SEX EDUCATION FOR TEENS

CRUSHING,

FLIRTING,

AND FIGURING IT ALL OUT...

SEX EDUCATION FOR TEENS

Crushing,
Flirting,
and Figuring It All Out...

Duke Firestone

Seattle
2024

4

Duke Firestone

Duke.Firestone@gmail.com

ISBN: 979-8879643664

First Edition

Seattle 2024

Macho House

To Teenagers

Contents

Preface

Dear Reader,

As I sit down to write this preface, I'm filled with a sense of profound responsibility and excitement. Responsibility because I understand the weight of the subject matter we're about to delve into – the world of sex education for teenagers. Excitement because I firmly believe in the transformative power of knowledge and education, especially when it comes to topics as crucial and often misunderstood as sexuality.

Sex Education for Teens: Crushing, Flirting, and Figuring It All Out is not just another book on the shelf. It's a labor of love, born out of years of experience, research, and dedication to improving the lives of young people. As a sexologist and educator, I've had the privilege of working with countless teenagers, witnessing their struggles, triumphs, and everything in between. And through it all, one thing has become abundantly clear – the need for comprehensive, inclusive, and empathetic sex education.

This book is my humble attempt to fill that need. It's a roadmap for teenagers navigating the often confusing and overwhelming world of relationships, desires, and sexual health. But it's also a celebration of diversity, empowerment, and self-discovery. Whether you're grappling with your first crush, exploring the nuances of flirting, or questioning your identity, this book is here to offer guidance, support, and understanding.

But let me be clear – this book is not just about imparting information. It's about fostering critical thinking, empathy, and respect. It's about empowering you to make informed decisions, set boundaries, and navigate the complexities of intimacy with confidence and agency. It's about creating a safe space where you can ask questions, share experiences, and learn from each other.

I want to thank you for embarking on this journey with me. Whether you're a teenager grappling with your own questions and uncertainties or an adult seeking to support the young people in your life, your presence here is invaluable. Together, let's embark on a journey of learning, growth, and self-discovery.

With warmest regards,
Duke Firestone

Introduction

Welcome to Sex Education for Teens.

In today's world, navigating the complexities of relationships, desires, and sexual health can be challenging, yet essential for your well-being and growth. This book is designed to be your trusted guide through this journey of self-discovery and understanding. Whether you're experiencing your first crush, exploring the realm of flirting, or grappling with questions about identity and intimacy, this book is here to provide you with the knowledge, tools, and support you need.

Why This Book Matters

Sex education is more than just learning about biology or reproductive health; it's about empowering you to make informed decisions, foster healthy relationships, and embrace your sexuality with confidence and respect. Unfortunately, many teens lack access to comprehensive and inclusive sex education, leaving them vulnerable to misinformation, shame, and uncertainty. This book aims to bridge that gap by offering a holistic approach to sex education that acknowledges the emotional, social, and cultural aspects of sexuality.

Understanding Your Journey

Embarking on the journey of adolescence is a transformative experience filled with excitement, curiosity, and sometimes confusion. As you navigate through this period of self-discovery, it's important to recognize that your journey is unique and valid. You may encounter challenges, setbacks, and moments of doubt along the way, but remember that you are not alone. This book is here to accompany you every step of the way, providing guidance, support, and encouragement as you navigate the intricacies of teenagehood and sexuality.

Together, let's embark on this journey of learning, growth, and self-discovery. Welcome to Sex Education for Teens..

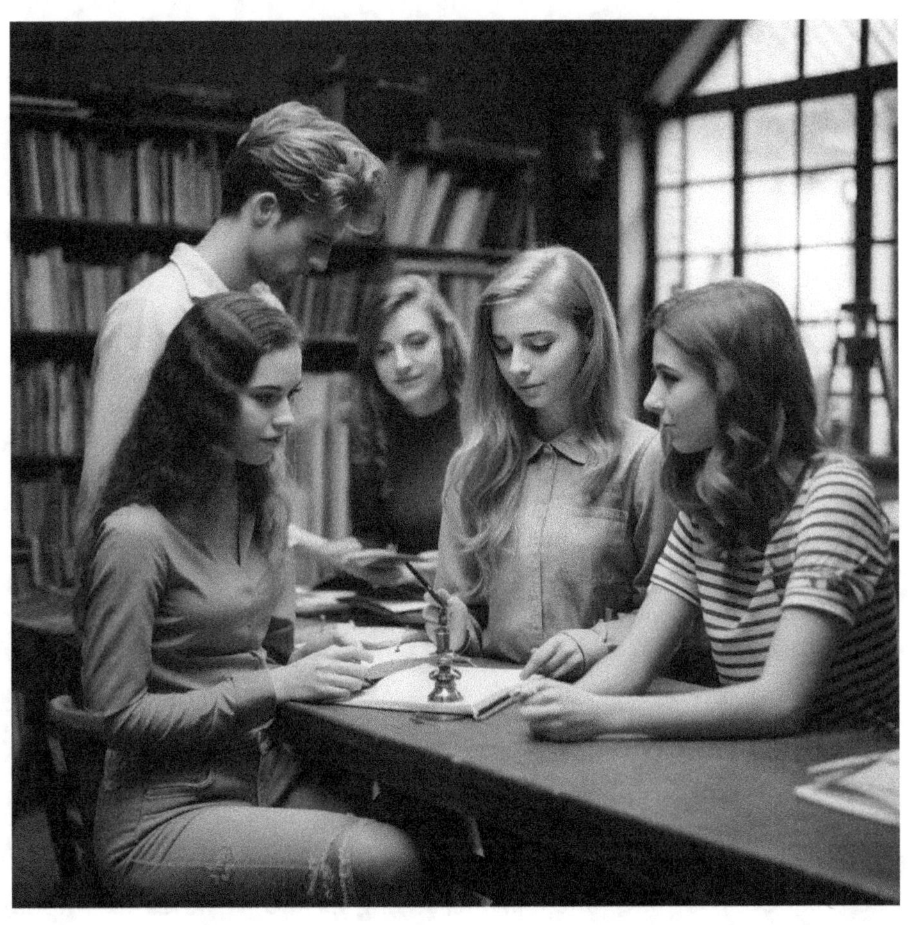

Chapter 1

Understanding Yourself

Welcome to the first chapter of Sex Education for Teens: Crushing, Flirting, and Figuring It All Out. In this chapter, we'll embark on a journey of self-discovery, starting with the exploration of your identity.

As a teenager, you're at a stage in life where you're constantly evolving, discovering new facets of yourself, and trying to make sense of the world around you. This process of self-exploration is not always easy. You may find yourself grappling with questions about who you are, what you believe in, and where you fit in society. And that's perfectly okay.

Identity is a multifaceted concept that encompasses various aspects of your being – your personality, interests, values, beliefs, and experiences. It's not something that can be easily defined or categorized. Instead, it's a fluid and dynamic construct that evolves over time.

One of the first steps in exploring your identity is to cultivate self-awareness – the ability to recognize and understand your thoughts, feelings, and behaviors. Take some time to reflect on what makes you unique – your likes and dislikes, strengths and weaknesses, hopes and dreams. Journaling, meditation, or simply engaging in introspective conversations with yourself can be helpful practices in this regard.

It's also important to recognize that identity is not fixed or predetermined. It's okay to experiment, try new things, and explore different aspects of yourself. Don't be afraid to step out of your comfort zone and embrace opportunities for growth and self-discovery.

As you embark on this journey of self-exploration, remember to be kind and compassionate to yourself. Embrace your quirks, celebrate your accomplishments, and acknowledge your struggles. You are a work in progress, and that's something to be proud of.

In the next sections of this chapter, we'll delve deeper into topics like body positivity and self-love, as well as emotions and mental health. But for now, take a moment to appreciate the unique individual that you are, and the exciting journey of self-discovery that lies ahead.

Now that we've begun our exploration of identity, let's turn our attention to another crucial aspect of self-discovery: body positivity and self-love.

In today's society, we're bombarded with messages about what our bodies should look like, how we should dress, and what constitutes beauty. These messages often promote unrealistic standards and can lead to feelings of insecurity, shame, and self-doubt, especially during adolescence when our bodies are undergoing significant changes.

But here's the truth: Your worth is not determined by your appearance. Your body is uniquely yours, and it deserves to be celebrated and cherished, regardless of its shape, size, or perceived flaws.

Body positivity is about embracing and accepting your body just as it is – imperfections and all. It's about recognizing that beauty comes in all shapes, sizes, and forms, and that true beauty radiates from within.

Practicing self-love is an essential part of cultivating body positivity. It involves treating yourself with kindness, compassion, and respect, both physically and emotionally. This means nourishing your body with nutritious food, getting enough rest, staying active, and engaging in activities that bring you joy and fulfillment.

But self-love goes beyond just taking care of your physical health. It's also about nurturing your mental and emotional well-being. This brings us to our next topic: emotions and mental health.

As a teenager, you're likely experiencing a wide range of emotions — from excitement and joy to sadness and anxiety. It's important to remember that all emotions are valid and normal, and it's okay to feel what you're feeling.

However, navigating these emotions can sometimes be challenging, especially when dealing with issues like peer pressure, academic stress, or family conflicts. That's why it's crucial to prioritize your mental health and seek support when needed.

This can include talking to a trusted friend or family member, reaching out to a school counselor or mental health professional, or practicing self-care activities like meditation, mindfulness, or creative expression.

Remember, you are not alone in your journey. There are people who care about you and want to support you. And by prioritizing your well-being and practicing self-love, you're taking an important step towards living a fulfilling and empowered life.

In the next section of this chapter, we'll delve deeper into emotions and mental health, exploring strategies for managing stress, building resilience, and fostering emotional well-being. But for now, take a moment to reflect on your own relationship with your body and emotions, and remember to be gentle and compassionate with yourself as you continue on your journey of self-discovery.

As we continue our exploration of identity, let's delve deeper into the importance of body positivity and self-love.

Body positivity is not just about accepting your physical appearance; it's about embracing your body as a whole – including its abilities, functions, and uniqueness. This means shifting your focus away from unrealistic beauty standards promoted by society and instead celebrating the diversity and individuality of bodies.

One way to foster body positivity is by practicing self-love. Self-love involves cultivating a positive and compassionate relationship with yourself, treating yourself with kindness and respect, and prioritizing your well-being. It means acknowledging your worthiness and deservingness of love and care, regardless of external validation.

Practicing self-love also entails recognizing and challenging negative self-talk and beliefs about your body. This might involve reframing negative thoughts into more positive and affirming ones, or engaging in activities that promote self-acceptance and appreciation.

Additionally, it's important to surround yourself with supportive and empowering influences that reinforce body positivity. Seek out communities, media, and role models that celebrate diverse bodies and promote messages of self-acceptance and self-love.

Now, let's shift our focus to emotions and mental health. As a teenager, you're likely experiencing a wide range of emotions as you navigate the ups and downs of adolescence. From the excitement of new experiences to the challenges of academic pressures and social dynamics, it's normal to feel a rollercoaster of emotions.

However, it's essential to recognize that your mental health matters just as much as your physical health. Mental health encompasses your emotional, psychological, and social well-being, and it plays a significant role in your overall quality of life.

Taking care of your mental health involves prioritizing self-care practices that promote emotional well-being, such as:

1. Practicing mindfulness and relaxation techniques to manage stress and anxiety.

2. Engaging in regular physical activity to boost mood and reduce symptoms of depression.

3. Cultivating supportive relationships and seeking help when needed.

4. Setting boundaries and prioritizing your needs and boundaries.

5. Finding healthy outlets for expression, such as journaling, art, or music.

Remember, it's okay to not be okay sometimes. Everyone experiences challenges and setbacks, and it's important to be gentle and compassionate with yourself during difficult times. If you're struggling with your mental health, don't hesitate to reach out for support from trusted friends, family members, or mental health professionals.

Emotions are an integral part of the human experience. They serve as signals, communicating important information about our internal state and external environment. As a teenager, you may find yourself experiencing a wide range of emotions — from happiness and excitement to sadness and anger. It's essential to recognize and validate these emotions, as they provide valuable insights into your needs, desires, and boundaries.

However, navigating emotions can sometimes be challenging, especially when faced with stressors such as academic pressures, peer conflicts, or family issues. That's where emotional intelligence comes into play.

Emotional intelligence refers to the ability to recognize, understand, and manage both your own emotions and the emotions of others. It involves skills such as self-awareness, self-regulation, empathy, and effective communication.

One way to enhance your emotional intelligence is by practicing mindfulness — the practice of being present and nonjudgmental of your thoughts, feelings, and sensations. Mindfulness can help you cultivate greater self-awareness, regulate your emotions more effectively, and develop a deeper understanding of yourself and others.

Additionally, building healthy coping mechanisms is essential for managing stress and maintaining emotional well-being. Healthy coping mechanisms may include:

- Engaging in physical activity, such as exercise or yoga, to release pent-up tension and boost mood.

- Practicing relaxation techniques, such as deep breathing or progressive muscle relaxation, to alleviate stress and anxiety.

- Seeking social support from friends, family members, or trusted adults when feeling overwhelmed or distressed.

- Engaging in hobbies and activities that bring joy and fulfillment, such as games, music, or spending time in nature.

It's important to remember that taking care of your mental health is not a sign of weakness but rather a sign of strength and resilience. Just as you would prioritize your physical health by eating nutritious foods and exercising regularly, it's equally important to prioritize your emotional well-being by practicing self-care and seeking support when needed.

Self-awareness is the ability to recognize and understand our thoughts, emotions, behaviors, and values. It involves introspection, reflection, and an honest appraisal of ourselves. Developing self-awareness is a lifelong journey that requires mindfulness and a willingness to explore our innermost thoughts and feelings.

One aspect of self-awareness is understanding our strengths and weaknesses. By acknowledging our strengths, we can build upon them to achieve our goals and aspirations. Similarly, recognizing our weaknesses allows us to identify areas for growth and improvement. Embracing both our strengths and weaknesses helps us cultivate a sense of authenticity and self-acceptance.

Another aspect of self-awareness is understanding our emotions. Emotions play a crucial role in shaping our experiences and interactions with the world around us. By becoming more aware of our emotions, we can better regulate them and respond to situations in a healthy and constructive manner. This includes recognizing triggers, understanding the underlying causes of our emotions, and developing effective coping strategies.

Additionally, self-awareness involves understanding our values and beliefs. Our values guide our decision-making process and shape our priorities in life. By clarifying our values, we can make choices that are aligned with our authentic selves and lead to greater fulfillment and purpose.

Cultivating self-awareness requires practice and patience. It involves regularly checking in with ourselves, engaging in self-reflection, and seeking feedback from others. Journaling, meditation, and mindfulness practices can also help deepen our self-awareness and enhance our understanding of ourselves.

Self-acceptance is the foundation upon which a healthy sense of self is built. It involves embracing all aspects of ourselves – our strengths and weaknesses, our successes and failures, our virtues and flaws. Self-acceptance means recognizing that we are worthy of love and respect, regardless of external validation or societal standards.

Practicing self-acceptance requires compassion and kindness towards ourselves. It means letting go of harsh self-judgments and unrealistic expectations, and instead, embracing our imperfections with humility and grace. Self-acceptance is not about complacency or resignation; rather, it's about acknowledging our humanity and striving to grow and evolve as individuals.

Self-expression is another vital component of understanding ourselves. It involves authentically expressing who we are – our thoughts, feelings, beliefs, and desires – in ways that are genuine and true to ourselves. Self-expression can take many forms, from artistic pursuits like writing, music, or painting, to more subtle forms like communication style and fashion choices.

Expressing ourselves authentically allows us to connect with others on a deeper level and cultivate meaningful relationships. It fosters a sense of belonging and validation, as we share our unique perspectives and experiences with the world. Self-expression is also a powerful tool for self-discovery, as it helps us clarify our values, aspirations, and sense of purpose.

However, self-expression can sometimes feel daunting, especially in a world that often values conformity over individuality. It takes courage to speak our truth and show up authentically in a society that may not always embrace our uniqueness. But the rewards of self-expression – authenticity, connection, and personal fulfillment – far outweigh the risks.

Values are the principles, standards, and ideals that are important to us and guide our behavior and decision-making. They represent what we believe to be right, meaningful, and worthy in life. Our values serve as a compass, helping us navigate the complexities of the world and make choices that are aligned with our authentic selves.

Identifying our values requires introspection and reflection. It involves examining our beliefs, priorities, and aspirations, and clarifying what truly matters to us. Our values may encompass a wide range of domains, including relationships, work, spirituality, personal growth, community, and social justice.

Once we have identified our values, it's essential to align our actions and choices with them. Living in accordance with our values brings a sense of integrity, purpose, and fulfillment to our lives. It allows us to lead lives that are meaningful and authentic, and to make decisions that are consistent with our deepest desires and aspirations.

However, living in alignment with our values can sometimes be challenging, especially in a world that may not always support or validate our beliefs. It requires courage, resilience, and a willingness to stand up for what we believe in, even in the face of opposition or adversity. But the rewards of living authentically and in accordance with our values — a sense of fulfillment, inner peace, and purpose — far outweigh the challenges.

In addition to values, our beliefs also play a significant role in shaping our identities and guiding our actions. Beliefs are the assumptions, convictions, and interpretations that we hold about ourselves, others, and the world around us. They influence our thoughts, feelings, and behaviors, and shape our perceptions of reality.

Our beliefs can be both empowering and limiting. Empowering beliefs support our growth, resilience, and well-being, while limiting beliefs can hold us back and prevent us from reaching our full potential.

Identifying and challenging limiting beliefs is essential for personal growth and development, as it allows us to break free from self-imposed barriers and live more fully and authentically.

In the next sections of this chapter, we will explore strategies for identifying our values and beliefs, aligning our actions with our values, and challenging limiting beliefs that may be holding us back. But for now, take a moment to reflect on your own values and beliefs. What principles and ideals are important to you? How do your values and beliefs shape your identity and guide your actions? By exploring these questions, you can gain greater insight into yourself and your journey of self-discovery.

Identifying our values is a deeply personal process that requires introspection and self-awareness. One way to begin this process is by reflecting on moments in your life when you felt truly fulfilled, satisfied, or aligned with your sense of purpose. What values were present in those moments? What principles were you upholding or pursuing? These reflections can provide valuable insights into the values that are most important to you.

Another approach to identifying your values is to consider what qualities you admire in others and aspire to embody in your own life. Think about the people you look up to – whether they're friends, family members, mentors, or public figures – and the characteristics that you admire in them. These qualities may offer clues about the values that resonate most deeply with you.

Once you have identified your values, it's essential to align your actions and choices with them. This requires mindfulness and intentionality in how you navigate your daily life. Ask yourself: Are my actions and decisions consistent with my values? Am I living in alignment with what truly matters to me? Making conscious choices that reflect your values can bring a greater sense of authenticity, purpose, and fulfillment to your life.

In addition to values, our beliefs also play a significant role in shaping our identities and guiding our actions. Beliefs are the lenses through which we interpret the world around us and make sense of our experiences. They influence our perceptions, attitudes, and behaviors, and can have a profound impact on our lives.

Some beliefs are empowering and supportive of our growth and well-being, while others may be limiting and hold us back from reaching our full potential. Identifying and challenging limiting beliefs is essential for personal growth and development. This may involve questioning the validity of our beliefs, examining the evidence that supports or contradicts them, and reframing them in a more empowering and constructive light.

Aligning our actions with our values requires ongoing reflection and conscious decision-making. It involves regularly assessing whether our behaviors and choices are in harmony with the principles and ideals that we hold dear. This may require making difficult decisions or stepping outside of our comfort zones to stay true to our values, even when it's not the easiest or most popular choice.

One helpful strategy for aligning our actions with our values is setting clear intentions and goals that reflect what matters most to us. By articulating our values and aspirations, we can create a roadmap for living in accordance with them and making choices that honor our deepest desires and principles.

Another important aspect of living in alignment with our values is practicing self-awareness and mindfulness in our daily lives. This means paying attention to our thoughts, feelings, and behaviors, and noticing when we may be acting in ways that are inconsistent with our values. By cultivating a greater awareness of our actions and their alignment with our values, we can make more intentional choices that reflect our authentic selves.

In addition to aligning our actions with our values, it's also essential to challenge limiting beliefs that may be holding us back from reaching our full potential. Limiting beliefs are often deeply ingrained and can manifest as negative self-talk, self-doubt, or fear of failure. They can undermine our confidence, resilience, and ability to pursue our goals and aspirations.

Challenging limiting beliefs involves questioning their validity and reframing them in a more empowering and constructive light. This may involve gathering evidence that contradicts the belief, seeking out alternative perspectives, and replacing negative self-talk with more supportive and encouraging language. By challenging limiting beliefs, we can create new narratives that empower us to overcome obstacles, take risks, and pursue our dreams with confidence and conviction.

One effective strategy for aligning our actions with our values is to create concrete action plans that reflect our values and goals. This involves breaking down our aspirations into smaller, manageable steps and identifying specific actions we can take to move closer to our desired outcomes. By translating our values into actionable behaviors, we can ensure that our daily actions are in line with what matters most to us.

Regular self-reflection is another valuable tool for staying aligned with our values. Taking time to reflect on our thoughts, feelings, and behaviors allows us to assess whether our actions are consistent with our values and identify areas where we may need to make adjustments. Journaling, meditation, or simply setting aside dedicated time for introspection can help us cultivate greater self-awareness and ensure that we're living in alignment with our deepest principles and ideals.

In addition to aligning our actions with our values, it's essential to challenge limiting beliefs that may be holding us back from realizing our full potential. One effective way to do this is through cognitive restructuring, a technique used in cognitive-behavioral therapy to challenge and reframe negative thought patterns. This involves identifying negative or self-defeating beliefs, examining the evidence that supports or contradicts them, and replacing them with more accurate and empowering beliefs.

For example, if you struggle with the belief that you're not good enough, you might challenge this belief by reflecting on past accomplishments and successes, seeking out supportive evidence from friends or loved ones, and reframing negative self-talk with more positive and affirming language. By consciously challenging and reframing limiting beliefs, we can create new narratives that support our growth, resilience, and well-being.

In conclusion, the journey of understanding yourself is an ongoing and deeply personal exploration that encompasses various dimensions of your identity, including your values, beliefs, emotions, and physical self. Through exploring your identity, cultivating body positivity and self-love, and prioritizing your emotional and mental well-being, you can cultivate a deeper sense of self-awareness, acceptance, and authenticity.

By embracing who you are, celebrating your unique qualities, and nurturing your physical, emotional, and mental health, you can embark on a journey of self-discovery and personal growth that leads to greater fulfillment, resilience, and well-being. Remember that authenticity is not about being perfect or conforming to others' expectations; it's about embracing your truth, honoring your values, and living in alignment with what matters most to you.

As you continue on your journey of understanding yourself, know that you are worthy of love, acceptance, and belonging just as you are. Embrace your strengths, acknowledge your vulnerabilities, and trust in your innate wisdom and intuition to guide you forward. By staying true to yourself and honoring your authentic voice, you can create a life that is rich in meaning, purpose, and fulfillment.

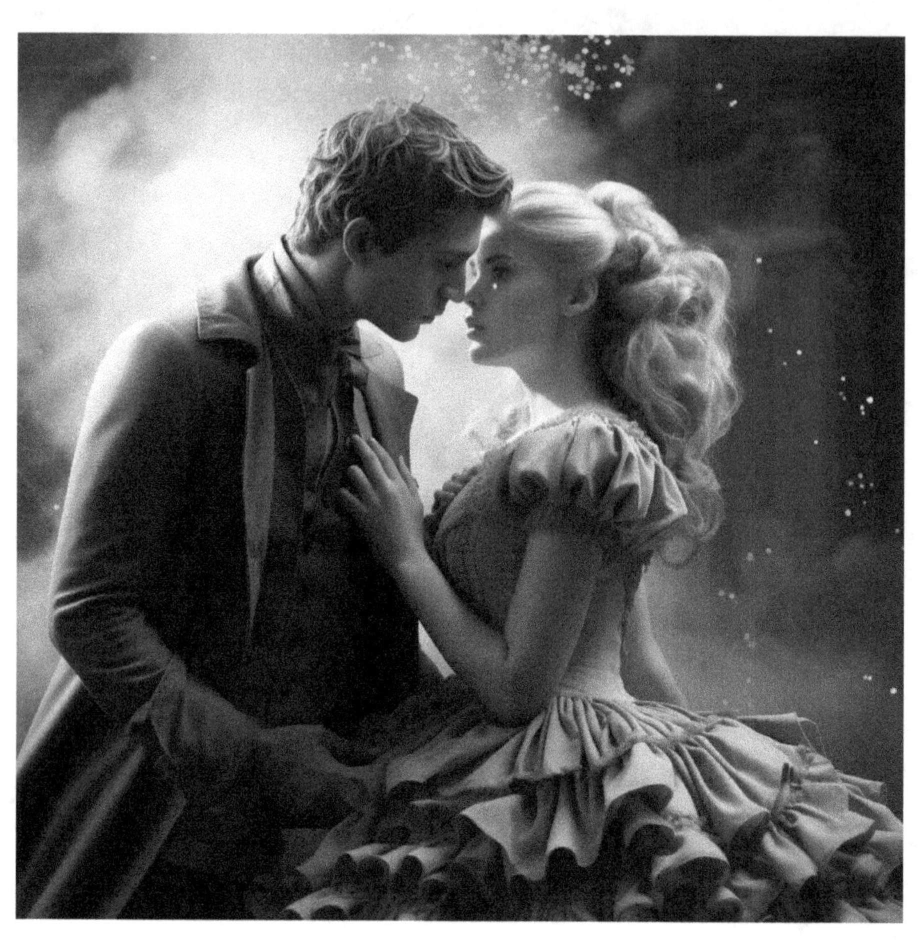

Chapter 2

Crushing 101

What is a Crush?

Ah, the exhilarating rush of a crush — a feeling that many of us have experienced at some point in our lives. But what exactly is a crush?

At its core, a crush is an intense and often fleeting infatuation or attraction towards someone else. It's that fluttery feeling in your stomach, the racing of your heart, and the incessant thoughts that occupy your mind when you're around that special someone. A crush can be sparked by physical attraction, personality traits, shared interests, or simply a mysterious and unexplainable connection.

But a crush is more than just a passing fancy; it's a complex blend of emotions, fantasies, and desires that can leave us feeling elated, anxious, and everything in between. It's a potent cocktail of excitement and uncertainty, as we navigate the exhilarating highs and nerve-wracking lows of infatuation.

What sets a crush apart from other forms of attraction is its often one-sided nature. While you may feel deeply drawn to someone, they may not necessarily reciprocate your feelings — at least not in the same way. This asymmetry can be both thrilling and agonizing, as we grapple with the uncertainty of whether our feelings will be returned.

Despite its inherent complexities and uncertainties, a crush can be a transformative experience that teaches us valuable lessons about ourselves and our relationships. It can awaken us to the depths of our emotions, challenge our assumptions and beliefs, and inspire us to step outside of our comfort zones in pursuit of love and connection.

In the pages that follow, we'll explore the nuances of crushing – from navigating the exhilarating highs to coping with the inevitable heartaches. We'll delve into the psychology of attraction, examine the role of hormones and neurotransmitters in fueling our infatuation, and offer practical tips for managing the rollercoaster ride of emotions that comes with crushing.

As we delve deeper into the intricacies of crushing, it's important to recognize that crushes come in various forms and can manifest in different ways for different people. While some crushes may be fleeting and superficial, others can develop into deeper connections and meaningful relationships over time.

One aspect of understanding crushes is recognizing the role of attraction – both physical and emotional. Physical attraction often serves as the initial spark that ignites a crush, drawing us in with someone's appearance, charm, or charisma. However, it's essential to remember that attraction goes beyond mere physical appearance; it also encompasses personality traits, shared interests, and emotional connections that deepen our infatuation.

Furthermore, crushes can be influenced by a myriad of factors, including social, cultural, and environmental influences. Our upbringing, peer group, and media portrayals of romance and relationships can all shape our perceptions of love and attraction, influencing who we develop crushes on and how we navigate those feelings.

Another key aspect of crushes is the role of fantasy and imagination. When we have a crush on someone, it's common to indulge in daydreams and fantasies about what a relationship with them might be like. These fantasies can be both exhilarating and comforting, offering a temporary escape from the uncertainties and complexities of real-life interactions.

However, it's important to approach crushes with a sense of mindfulness and self-awareness. While crushes can be thrilling and exhilarating, they can also be accompanied by feelings of insecurity, jealousy, and anxiety. It's essential to recognize and acknowledge these emotions, as well as the potential impact of our actions on ourselves and others.

One of the intriguing aspects of crushes is their fluidity – they can wax and wane, intensify and fade, sometimes without warning or explanation. What may start as a fleeting infatuation can develop into a deeper connection, while other crushes may fizzle out as quickly as they ignited. Understanding the ebb and flow of crushes can help us navigate the complexities of these feelings with greater ease and self-awareness.

Moreover, crushes can serve as powerful catalysts for personal growth and self-discovery. As we navigate the emotions and uncertainties of infatuation, we may uncover hidden desires, confront limiting beliefs, and explore new aspects of ourselves. Crushes can push us outside of our comfort zones, encouraging us to take risks, embrace vulnerability, and pursue the things that truly matter to us.

However, it's essential to approach crushes with a sense of mindfulness and perspective. While crushes can be exhilarating and transformative, they can also be accompanied by feelings of longing, frustration, and disappointment. It's important to recognize that crushes are just one aspect of our emotional landscape and not necessarily indicative of our worth or value as individuals.

Furthermore, crushes can sometimes blur the boundaries of platonic and romantic relationships, leading to complexities and ambiguities in our interactions with others. It's crucial to communicate openly and honestly with ourselves and others about our feelings and intentions, respecting boundaries and consent every step of the way.

Crushes, with their whirlwind of emotions and fantasies, can significantly influence our emotional state. The intensity of infatuation can lead to heightened emotions, ranging from euphoria and excitement to anxiety and insecurity. It's essential to recognize and acknowledge these feelings, allowing ourselves to experience them fully while also maintaining perspective and self-awareness.

Moreover, crushes can sometimes disrupt our existing relationships, particularly if we're in a committed partnership. It's natural to experience attraction to others, even when we're in a loving and fulfilling relationship. However, it's crucial to handle these feelings with care and integrity, communicating openly and honestly with our partners about our experiences and maintaining boundaries that uphold the trust and respect in our relationship.

Additionally, crushes can provide valuable opportunities for self-reflection and personal growth. As we navigate the complexities of infatuation, we may uncover deeper desires, fears, and insecurities that have been lying beneath the surface. Exploring these inner landscapes can lead to greater self-awareness and self-acceptance, ultimately contributing to our overall well-being and fulfillment.

However, it's essential to approach crushes with a sense of mindfulness and discernment. While the excitement of infatuation can be intoxicating, it's crucial to maintain a realistic perspective and avoid getting swept away by fantasies and idealizations. Taking time to ground ourselves in the present moment, practice self-care, and nurture our existing relationships can help us navigate crushes with greater clarity and integrity.

- **Dos:**

  - **Acknowledge Your Feelings**: It's important to recognize and validate your emotions when you develop a crush. Allow yourself to experience the full range of feelings that come with infatuation, from excitement and butterflies to vulnerability and uncertainty.

  - **Maintain Perspective**: While crushes can feel all-consuming, it's essential to maintain perspective and recognize that they are just one aspect of your life. Remember to prioritize your well-being, goals, and existing relationships, and avoid getting swept away by fantasies or idealizations.

  - **Communicate Openly and Honestly**: If appropriate, consider sharing your feelings with the person you have a crush on. Be honest and respectful in your communication, expressing your interest or admiration without putting pressure on them to reciprocate. However, also be prepared for the possibility of rejection and respect their boundaries and feelings.

  - **Focus on Self-Improvement**: Use the energy and motivation that comes with infatuation as an opportunity for personal growth and self-improvement. Invest in activities that bring you joy, pursue your passions, and work towards your goals, regardless of whether they involve your crush.

- o **Maintain Boundaries**: While it's natural to feel drawn to someone you have a crush on, it's essential to respect their boundaries and autonomy. Avoid crossing personal or emotional boundaries, and prioritize consent and mutual respect in your interactions.

- **Don'ts:**

  - o **Obsess Over Every Interaction**: It's easy to overanalyze every interaction with your crush, reading too much into their words or actions. Remember that people are complex, and their behavior may not always reflect your interpretations or expectations.

  - o **Stalk or Invade Privacy**: Resist the temptation to engage in behaviors that invade your crush's privacy or make them feel uncomfortable. Avoid excessive social media monitoring, lurking, or showing up uninvited in their personal spaces.

  - o **Put Your Life on Hold**: While it's natural to feel consumed by thoughts of your crush, avoid putting your life on hold or neglecting your responsibilities and commitments. Maintain a healthy balance between your personal life, relationships, and pursuit of your goals and aspirations.

  - o **Pursue Unavailable Individuals**: If your crush is already in a committed relationship or has made it clear that they're not interested, respect their boundaries and refrain from pursuing them further. Redirect your energy towards people who are available and receptive to your affection.

- o **Ignore Your Own Needs and Boundaries**: Don't sacrifice your own well-being or compromise your values and boundaries in pursuit of your crush. Prioritize self-care, set healthy boundaries, and advocate for your own needs and desires in all your interactions.

By following these dos and don'ts, you can navigate the complexities of crushes with integrity, respect, and self-awareness, ultimately fostering healthier and more fulfilling connections with others.

Crush Culture: Navigating Social Media and Peer Influence

In today's digital age, crushes are often influenced and amplified by social media and peer culture. Navigating the complexities of crushes in a hyperconnected world can present unique challenges, but with mindfulness and self-awareness, it's possible to maintain a healthy relationship with technology and peer influence.

1. **Social Media Boundaries**: Social media platforms offer unprecedented access to information about our crushes, from their daily activities to their personal interests and relationships. While it can be tempting to obsessively monitor their online presence, it's important to set boundaries and limit your exposure to triggers that may fuel unhealthy fixation or comparison.

2. **Authenticity Over Perception**: In the age of curated online personas and filtered images, it's easy to fall into the trap of comparing ourselves to others and feeling inadequate. Remember that social media often presents a distorted view of reality, and prioritize authenticity over perception. Focus

on cultivating genuine connections and self-expression rather than seeking validation or approval from others.

3. **Peer Pressure and Influence**: Peer culture can also play a significant role in shaping our perceptions of attraction and relationships. Whether it's pressure to conform to societal beauty standards or to pursue certain individuals based on peer approval, it's essential to resist the influence of external expectations and stay true to your own values and desires.

4. **Healthy Communication**: Instead of relying solely on social media or peer influence to navigate your crushes, prioritize direct and healthy communication. Engage in open and honest conversations with your crushes, expressing your feelings and intentions with integrity and respect. Avoid relying on passive-aggressive tactics or indirect communication methods, as they can lead to misunderstandings and misinterpretations.

5. **Mindful Consumption**: Be mindful of the content you consume on social media and the impact it has on your mental and emotional well-being. Consider curating your social media feeds to include content that uplifts and inspires you, rather than fuels comparison or negative self-talk. Practice self-care by taking breaks from social media when needed and engaging in activities that nourish your soul and spirit.

By navigating social media and peer influence with mindfulness and self-awareness, you can maintain a healthy relationship with technology and external pressures while fostering authentic connections and relationships in your life. Remember to prioritize your own well-being and values, and don't be afraid to seek support from trusted friends, family members, or mental health professionals if needed.

"Crushing 101" is an insightful exploration into the intricate world of crushes, offering practical guidance and insights for navigating the exhilarating yet often perplexing experiences of infatuation and attraction. The chapter begins by defining what a crush truly is, delving into its essence as a fleeting yet intense fascination with another person, fueled by a mix of physical attraction, emotional connection, and fantasy.

As the chapter progresses, it provides readers with valuable dos and don'ts for dealing with crushes. Dos include acknowledging and validating one's feelings, maintaining healthy communication, and prioritizing personal growth and self-improvement. On the other hand, don'ts caution against obsessive behaviors, invading privacy, and pursuing individuals who are unavailable or uninterested.

Furthermore, "Crushing 101" examines the influence of social media and peer culture on crushes. In today's digital age, crushes are often amplified and shaped by social media platforms and peer dynamics. The chapter explores strategies for navigating this crush culture, emphasizing the importance of setting boundaries, prioritizing authenticity, and fostering offline connections.

In essence, "Crushing 101" serves as a comprehensive guide for readers to understand, navigate, and thrive amidst the complexities of crushes. By providing practical advice, insights, and reflections, the chapter equips readers with the tools they need to navigate the exhilarating journey of infatuation with grace, integrity, and self-awareness.

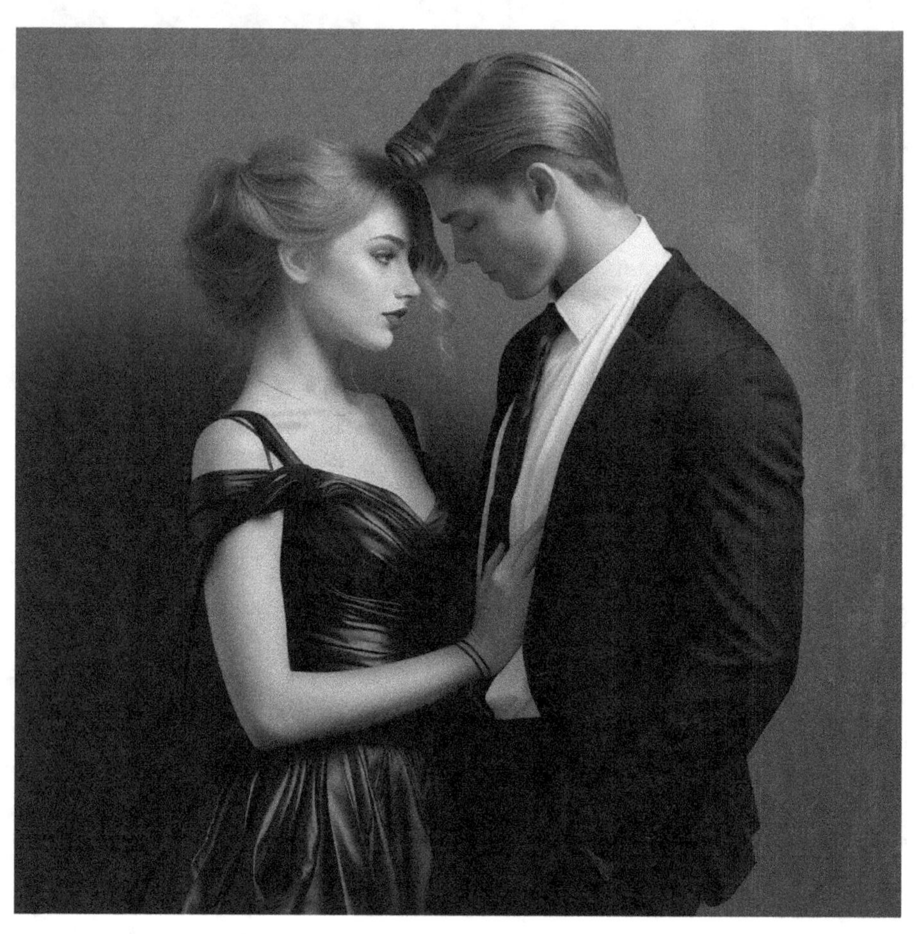

Chapter 3

Flirting with Confidence

Welcome to the exciting world of flirting! In this chapter, we'll explore the art of flirting, a skill that can add joy, excitement, and connection to your interactions with others. Whether you're looking to spark a romantic interest, build rapport with a new acquaintance, or simply enjoy playful banter, mastering the art of flirting can enhance your social interactions and relationships.

The Art of Flirting:

Flirting is a subtle and nuanced form of communication that involves expressing interest, attraction, and playfulness towards someone you're drawn to. It's a dance of wit, charm, and body language that conveys your intentions and creates a sense of rapport and chemistry. While flirting is often associated with romantic or sexual interest, it can also be a lighthearted and enjoyable way to connect with others on a platonic level.

At its core, the art of flirting is about creating positive and enjoyable interactions that leave both parties feeling valued, respected, and uplifted. It's about building rapport, fostering connection, and creating moments of shared laughter and enjoyment. While flirting can vary in intensity and context, from subtle gestures to more overt expressions of interest, the underlying principles remain the same: authenticity, confidence, and respect.

Throughout this chapter, we'll explore various tips, techniques, and strategies for mastering the art of flirting with confidence and authenticity. From body language cues to playful banter, we'll delve into the nuances of flirting and offer practical advice for enhancing your skills and creating meaningful connections with others. So, get ready to unleash your inner flirt and embark on a journey of playful interaction and connection!

Flirting is an intricate dance of communication that involves subtle cues, playful banter, and genuine interest. To master this art, it's essential to understand the nuances and techniques that make flirting effective and enjoyable. Here are some tips to help you become a confident and charismatic flirt:

1. **Body Language**: Pay attention to your body language as it can convey a lot about your intentions and feelings. Maintain open and relaxed postures, make eye contact, and use subtle gestures like smiling and leaning in to show interest and engagement.

2. **Initiate Light Touch**: When appropriate, incorporate light and playful touches into your interactions. A gentle touch on the arm or shoulder can create a sense of intimacy and connection, but be mindful of personal boundaries and comfort levels.

3. **Engage in Banter**: Playful banter is a hallmark of flirting and can keep conversations light and entertaining. Tease gently, exchange witty remarks, and maintain a playful tone to create a sense of rapport and chemistry.

4. **Active Listening**: Show genuine interest in the other person by actively listening to what they have to say. Ask open-ended questions, nod in agreement, and provide thoughtful responses to demonstrate your engagement and appreciation.

5. **Sincere Compliments**: Offer sincere compliments that highlight the other person's qualities or accomplishments. Be specific and genuine in your praise, and avoid overly generic or superficial compliments.

6. **Create Intrigue**: Leave a little mystery and intrigue to keep the other person curious and interested. Avoid revealing everything about yourself upfront and instead, share snippets of your personality and interests to invite further conversation and connection.

7. **Confidence and Authenticity**: Confidence is attractive, so own your unique qualities and quirks with pride. Be authentic and genuine in your interactions, and don't be afraid to show vulnerability or share personal stories—it can deepen the connection and foster intimacy.

8. **Respect Boundaries**: While flirting can be fun and exciting, it's important to respect the other person's boundaries and comfort levels. Pay attention to their verbal and non-verbal cues, and know when to dial back the intensity or take a step back if they seem uncomfortable.

By incorporating these tips and techniques into your flirting repertoire, you can enhance your social interactions, build meaningful connections, and enjoy the thrill of playful banter and genuine connection. So, embrace your inner flirt and have fun exploring the art of flirting!

Body language is a powerful tool in the art of flirting, capable of conveying a myriad of messages without uttering a single word. By mastering the subtleties of body language, you can enhance your ability to connect with others, express interest, and build rapport in social interactions. Here are some key aspects of body language to keep in mind when flirting:

1. **Maintain Open and Relaxed Postures:** Your posture speaks volumes about your confidence and comfort level. Avoid crossing your arms or legs, as this can signal defensiveness or disinterest. Instead, opt for open and

relaxed postures that convey approachability and receptiveness. Stand or sit up straight, with your shoulders back and your chest open, to exude confidence and warmth.

2. **Make Eye Contact**: Eye contact is a powerful form of nonverbal communication that can create a sense of connection and intimacy. When flirting, make a concerted effort to maintain steady eye contact with the other person. This shows that you are engaged and interested in what they have to say, and it can also convey confidence and sincerity. However, be mindful not to stare intently, as this can come across as aggressive or intimidating. Instead, aim for a natural and relaxed gaze that feels comfortable for both parties.

3. **Use Subtle Gestures**: Subtle gestures can add depth and nuance to your interactions, helping to convey interest and engagement. A genuine smile can instantly brighten your face and signal warmth and friendliness. Leaning in slightly towards the other person can create a sense of intimacy and closeness, while nodding in agreement can show that you are actively listening and engaged in the conversation. Pay attention to the other person's body language as well, and mirror their gestures and movements to create a sense of rapport and connection.

4. **Be Mindful of Personal Space**: Personal space is an important aspect of body language that can vary depending on cultural norms and individual preferences. When flirting, be mindful of the other person's personal space and respect their boundaries. Avoid standing too close or invading their personal space without invitation, as this can feel intrusive or uncomfortable. Instead, maintain a comfortable distance and gauge their reactions to ensure that you are both on the same page.

In summary, mastering the art of body language is essential for successful flirting. By maintaining open and relaxed postures, making eye contact, using subtle gestures, and respecting personal space, you can convey interest, warmth, and sincerity in your interactions. So, next time you find yourself flirting with someone special, remember to let your body do the talking!

In the intricate dance of flirting, incorporating light and playful touches can add a layer of intimacy and connection to your interactions. When executed appropriately, a gentle touch on the arm or shoulder can convey warmth, interest, and affection, creating a memorable moment of connection between you and the other person. However, it's crucial to approach physical touch with mindfulness and respect for personal boundaries.

Here are some key considerations to keep in mind when initiating light touch:

1. **Read the Situation**: Before initiating any form of physical touch, take a moment to assess the context and dynamics of the interaction. Is the other person receptive to your advances? Are they displaying signs of comfort and engagement? Pay attention to their body language and verbal cues to gauge their level of interest and comfort.

2. **Choose the Right Moment**: Timing is everything when it comes to initiating physical touch. Look for opportune moments during the conversation where a light touch would feel natural and appropriate. For example, if the other person shares something personal or funny, a light touch on the arm or shoulder can serve as a gesture of support or camaraderie.

3. **Start Small**: When initiating physical touch, start with small and subtle gestures before escalating to more intimate forms of contact. A light touch on the forearm or upper arm is

generally well-received and can convey interest and affection without being overly intrusive. Pay attention to the other person's reaction and adjust your approach accordingly.

4. **Be Mindful of Personal Boundaries**: While physical touch can enhance connection and intimacy, it's essential to respect the other person's personal boundaries and comfort levels. If they recoil or seem uncomfortable with your touch, immediately apologize and refrain from initiating further contact. Everyone has different preferences when it comes to physical touch, so it's crucial to prioritize consent and respect at all times.

5. **Pay Attention to Feedback:** As you initiate light touch, pay close attention to the other person's reactions and cues. Are they reciprocating your gestures? Do they seem to enjoy the physical contact, or do they appear uncomfortable? Adjust your approach based on their feedback, and be prepared to back off if your advances are not well-received.

In summary, initiating light touch can be a powerful way to create a sense of intimacy and connection in your interactions. By approaching physical touch with mindfulness, respect, and sensitivity to personal boundaries, you can enhance the quality of your flirting and deepen your connections with others in meaningful and memorable ways. So, the next time you're flirting with someone special, don't be afraid to reach out and make a gentle connection— it could be the start of something truly magical.

Banter is the lifeblood of flirting, injecting conversations with energy, humor, and spontaneity. When done effectively, playful banter can create a delightful back-and-forth exchange that fosters a sense of rapport and chemistry between you and the other person. By teasing gently, exchanging witty remarks, and maintaining a playful tone, you can infuse your interactions with excitement and intrigue.

Here are some tips for engaging in banter:

1. **Keep it Light and Lighthearted**: Banter is all about keeping things fun and enjoyable. Avoid heavy or sensitive topics that could dampen the mood or create tension. Instead, focus on lighthearted subjects that invite laughter and playfulness.

2. **Tease Gently**: Teasing is a central component of banter, but it's essential to do so in a gentle and good-natured manner. Avoid making overly personal or hurtful remarks, and always be mindful of the other person's feelings. The goal is to evoke smiles and laughter, not to offend or upset.

3. **Exchange Witty Remarks**: Quick wit and clever comebacks are the currency of banter. Keep your responses sharp and witty, and don't be afraid to engage in friendly verbal sparring. A well-timed quip or clever retort can keep the conversation flowing and leave both parties eagerly anticipating the next exchange.

4. **Maintain a Playful Tone**: The tone of your banter sets the stage for the interaction. Keep things light, playful, and upbeat, and avoid taking yourself too seriously. Embrace a spirit of spontaneity and adventure, and allow yourself to let loose and have fun with the conversation.

5. **Pay Attention to the Other Person's Responses**: Banter is a two-way street, so pay close attention to the other person's reactions and responses. Are they laughing and smiling, or do they seem uncomfortable or disengaged? Adjust your approach based on their cues, and be prepared to dial back or ramp up the banter accordingly.

In summary, engaging in banter is an essential skill for flirting and building connections with others. By keeping things light and lighthearted, teasing gently, exchanging witty remarks, and maintaining a playful tone, you can create an enjoyable and memorable interaction that leaves both parties wanting more. So, embrace the art of playful conversation and let the banter flow!

Active Listening: The Key to Meaningful Connection

In the world of flirting, active listening is a powerful tool for building rapport, fostering understanding, and demonstrating genuine interest in the other person. By showing that you are fully present and engaged in the conversation, you can create a sense of connection and appreciation that enhances the quality of your interactions. Here's how to practice active listening effectively:

1. **Be Fully Present**: To engage in active listening, it's essential to be fully present in the moment and give the other person your undivided attention. Put away distractions such as your phone or other electronic devices, and focus on the person in front of you. Maintain eye contact and use nonverbal cues such as nodding and leaning in to show that you are actively listening and engaged in the conversation.

2. **Ask Open-Ended Questions**: Open-ended questions are a powerful way to encourage the other person to share more about themselves and their experiences. Instead of asking yes or no questions, ask questions that invite the other person to elaborate and share their thoughts and feelings. For example, instead of asking, "Did you have a good day?" you could ask, "What was the best part of your day?"

3. **Nod in Agreement**: Nodding in agreement is a simple yet effective way to show that you are actively listening and engaged in the conversation. It signals to the other person

that you are on the same page and that you value what they have to say. However, be sure to nod naturally and authentically, rather than overdoing it or nodding excessively.

4. **Provide Thoughtful Responses**: When the other person is speaking, take the time to listen carefully and process what they are saying before responding. Offer thoughtful responses that demonstrate your understanding and appreciation of their perspective. Reflect back on what they have said, and validate their feelings and experiences. For example, you could say, "That sounds like it was really challenging for you. I admire your resilience in handling that situation."

5. **Show Empathy and Understanding**: Active listening is not just about hearing the words that are spoken—it's also about understanding the emotions and underlying messages behind those words. Show empathy and understanding towards the other person's experiences and feelings, and validate their emotions without judgment or criticism. Let them know that you are there to support and listen to them, no matter what.

In summary, active listening is a foundational skill for successful flirting and building meaningful connections with others. By being fully present, asking open-ended questions, nodding in agreement, providing thoughtful responses, and showing empathy and understanding, you can create an environment of trust and appreciation that enriches your interactions and fosters deeper connections. So, the next time you're flirting with someone special, remember to listen actively and show genuine interest in what they have to say—it can make all the difference in building a lasting connection.

Complimenting Sincerely: The Art of Genuine Appreciation

In the realm of flirting, offering sincere compliments is a powerful way to express admiration, appreciation, and interest in the other person. However, it's crucial to deliver compliments thoughtfully and genuinely, focusing on qualities or accomplishments that resonate with you on a personal level. Here's how to master the art of sincere complimenting:

1. **Focus on Genuine Praise**: When offering a compliment, aim to highlight qualities or accomplishments that genuinely impress or inspire you. Whether it's their sense of humor, creativity, kindness, or intelligence, choose compliments that reflect your authentic appreciation and admiration for who they are as a person.

2. **Avoid Generic Compliments**: Generic compliments can come across as insincere or superficial, lacking the personal touch that makes compliments meaningful. Instead of resorting to clichés or platitudes, take the time to notice specific traits or actions that stand out to you and tailor your compliments accordingly. This shows that you've taken the time to observe and appreciate the other person for who they truly are.

3. **Steer Clear of Overly Sexualized Compliments**: While it's natural to feel attracted to someone and want to express your admiration, it's essential to avoid compliments that are overly sexualized or objectifying. Focus on complimenting the person's character, talents, or achievements rather than their physical appearance. This demonstrates respect and appreciation for the person as a whole, beyond just their outward appearance.

4. **Be Sincere and Authentic**: Sincerity is key when delivering compliments. Make sure your praise comes from a genuine place of admiration and respect, rather than an attempt to flatter or manipulate the other person. Be authentic in your words and delivery, and let your sincerity shine through in your tone and demeanor.

5. **Offer Compliments Sparingly**: While compliments can be a wonderful way to make someone feel appreciated and valued, it's essential to offer them sparingly and with discretion. Too many compliments can come across as insincere or overwhelming, so choose your moments wisely and focus on quality over quantity.

In summary, offering sincere compliments is a powerful way to express admiration, appreciation, and interest in the other person. By focusing on genuine praise, avoiding generic or overly sexualized compliments, being sincere and authentic in your delivery, and offering compliments sparingly and with discretion, you can master the art of sincere complimenting and create meaningful connections with others in your flirting endeavors. So, the next time you're drawn to someone special, don't hesitate to let them know what you genuinely appreciate about them—it could be the start of something beautiful.

Creating Intrigue: The Art of Mystery and Allure

In the realm of flirting, creating intrigue is like weaving a captivating story that leaves the other person eager to learn more about you. By strategically revealing parts of yourself while leaving other aspects shrouded in mystery, you can cultivate a sense of curiosity and anticipation that deepens the connection and keeps the conversation engaging. Here's how to master the art of creating intrigue:

1. **Reveal Strategically**: Instead of laying all your cards on the table upfront, reveal aspects of yourself gradually and strategically. Share anecdotes, insights, and experiences that offer glimpses into who you are, but leave enough unsaid to keep the other person intrigued and wanting to learn more.

2. **Sprinkle Hints and Clues**: Drop subtle hints and clues about your interests, passions, and quirks throughout your conversations. These hints serve as breadcrumbs that invite the other person to explore and discover more about you over time. Whether it's mentioning a favorite book, hobby, or travel destination, these hints can spark curiosity and conversation.

3. **Keep Them Guessing**: Embrace a sense of mystery and allure by keeping some aspects of yourself hidden from plain view. Avoid divulging too much personal information too soon, and instead, maintain an air of mystery that piques the other person's curiosity. Let them wonder about the depths of your personality and the secrets you have yet to reveal.

4. **Encourage Exploration**: Invite the other person to ask questions and delve deeper into your world. Encourage curiosity and exploration by being open to discussing various topics and sharing more about yourself as the conversation progresses. By inviting them to take an active role in uncovering the layers of your personality, you create opportunities for deeper connection and understanding.

5. **Maintain a Sense of Intrigue**: As the conversation unfolds, continue to sprinkle hints and clues that keep the other person guessing. Share anecdotes, experiences, and insights that reveal different facets of your personality, but always leave something left unsaid to maintain a sense of intrigue and mystery.

In summary, creating intrigue is an artful dance of revealing and concealing, enticing the other person to explore the depths of your personality and discover the hidden gems within. By strategically revealing parts of yourself while leaving other aspects shrouded in mystery, you can cultivate a sense of curiosity and anticipation that deepens the connection and keeps the conversation engaging. So, embrace the allure of mystery and let the other person be drawn into the captivating story of who you are.

Confidence is undeniably attractive, but true magnetism comes from authenticity. When you confidently own your strengths, quirks, and vulnerabilities, you radiate a genuine charisma that draws others in and fosters deep connections. Here's how to cultivate confidence and authenticity in your interactions:

1. **Own Your Strengths**: Recognize and celebrate your unique qualities, talents, and accomplishments. Whether you're passionate about a particular hobby, excel in a certain skill, or possess a natural charisma, embrace these strengths with pride. Confidence stems from acknowledging and appreciating the value you bring to the table.

2. **Embrace Your Quirks**: Your quirks and idiosyncrasies are what make you uniquely you. Instead of trying to fit into a mold of perceived perfection, embrace your quirks with humor and acceptance. Your authenticity will shine through when you're unapologetically yourself, quirks and all.

3. **Be Genuine**: Authenticity is magnetic. Be genuine in your interactions, expressing your thoughts, feelings, and opinions sincerely and without pretense. People are drawn to those who are unafraid to be themselves and speak from the heart.

4. **Show Vulnerability**: Vulnerability is not a sign of weakness but rather a display of courage and authenticity. Don't be

afraid to share your fears, insecurities, and struggles with others. Opening up about your vulnerabilities creates opportunities for empathy, understanding, and deeper connection.

5. **Share Personal Stories**: Personal stories are windows into your soul. Share your experiences, triumphs, and challenges with others, allowing them to see the layers of your personality and the depth of your character. Sharing personal stories fosters intimacy and strengthens bonds between individuals.

6. **Stay True to Yourself**: In a world that often pressures us to conform, staying true to yourself can be a revolutionary act. Trust in your instincts, values, and beliefs, and don't compromise them for the sake of others' approval. When you authentically express who you are, you attract like-minded individuals who appreciate you for you.

In summary, confidence and authenticity go hand in hand, creating a powerful synergy that draws others to you and fosters deep, meaningful connections. By owning your strengths and quirks with pride, being genuine in your interactions, showing vulnerability, sharing personal stories, and staying true to yourself, you cultivate an irresistible charm that captivates those around you. So, embrace your true self and let your authenticity shine brightly for the world to see.

Know When to Pull Back: Respecting Boundaries in Flirting

Flirting can be an exhilarating dance of attraction and connection, but it's important to remember that boundaries matter. Being attuned to the other person's signals and comfort levels is essential for creating a positive and respectful interaction. Here's how to navigate the delicate balance of knowing when to pull back:

1. **Pay Attention to Signals**: Communication goes beyond words, and it's crucial to pay attention to the other person's nonverbal cues and body language. Are they leaning in and maintaining eye contact, or are they shifting away and avoiding eye contact? These signals can provide valuable insight into their level of interest and comfort.

2. **Respect Comfort Levels**: Everyone has different comfort levels when it comes to flirting and physical contact. Respect the other person's boundaries and comfort zones, and avoid pushing them beyond their limits. If they seem hesitant or uncomfortable with a particular interaction, dial back the intensity and give them space to breathe.

3. **Be Mindful of Verbal Cues**: Verbal cues can also offer clues about the other person's feelings and boundaries. Listen for cues such as hesitancy, reluctance, or explicit statements of discomfort. If they express discomfort or disinterest, take their words seriously and adjust your behavior accordingly.

4. **Take a Step Back if Necessary**: If you sense that the other person is uninterested or uncomfortable, it's essential to take a step back and reassess the situation. Respect their boundaries and give them the space they need to feel comfortable and at ease. Remember that consent is paramount, and it's better to err on the side of caution than to push someone beyond their comfort zone.

5. **Communicate Openly**: If you're unsure about the other person's boundaries or comfort levels, don't hesitate to communicate openly and ask for clarification. Respectfully inquire about their preferences and comfort zones, and be receptive to their feedback. Open and honest communication is key to fostering trust and respect in any interaction.

6. **Know When to End the Interaction**: Sometimes, despite your best efforts to respect boundaries, the other person may still feel uncomfortable or uninterested. In such cases, know when to gracefully end the interaction and part ways amicably. Respect their decision and avoid pressuring them into further interaction.

In summary, knowing when to pull back is an essential skill in flirting and building healthy relationships. By paying attention to the other person's signals and boundaries, respecting their comfort levels, and communicating openly and honestly, you can create a positive and respectful interaction that honors both parties' needs and boundaries. So, the next time you're flirting with someone special, remember to tread lightly, listen attentively, and respect their boundaries every step of the way.

In the intricate dance of flirting, navigating the nuances of communication, connection, and boundaries is essential. Throughout this chapter, we've explored various aspects of flirting, from body language and banter to authenticity and respecting boundaries. By mastering these skills, you can enhance your interactions, deepen connections, and create meaningful relationships built on mutual respect and understanding.

Remember, flirting is not just about attracting someone's attention or winning them over—it's about fostering genuine connection, respect, and appreciation for the other person as an individual. Whether you're exchanging playful banter, sharing personal stories, or showing vulnerability, approach flirting with sincerity, authenticity, and a genuine desire to connect.

As you continue on your flirting journey, keep in mind the importance of listening attentively, respecting boundaries, and knowing when to pull back if the other person seems uncomfortable or uninterested. By prioritizing mutual respect and communication, you can create positive and enriching interactions that leave a lasting impression.

So, embrace the art of flirting with confidence, authenticity, and respect, and let your interactions be guided by sincerity, empathy, and genuine connection. Whether you're sparking a new romance or deepening an existing connection, may your flirting endeavors be filled with joy, excitement, and meaningful connections.

With that, we conclude this chapter on flirting, but the journey of self-discovery and connection continues. Stay tuned for the next chapter, where we'll delve into the exciting world of relationships and intimacy. Until then, may your interactions be filled with laughter, warmth, and genuine connection.

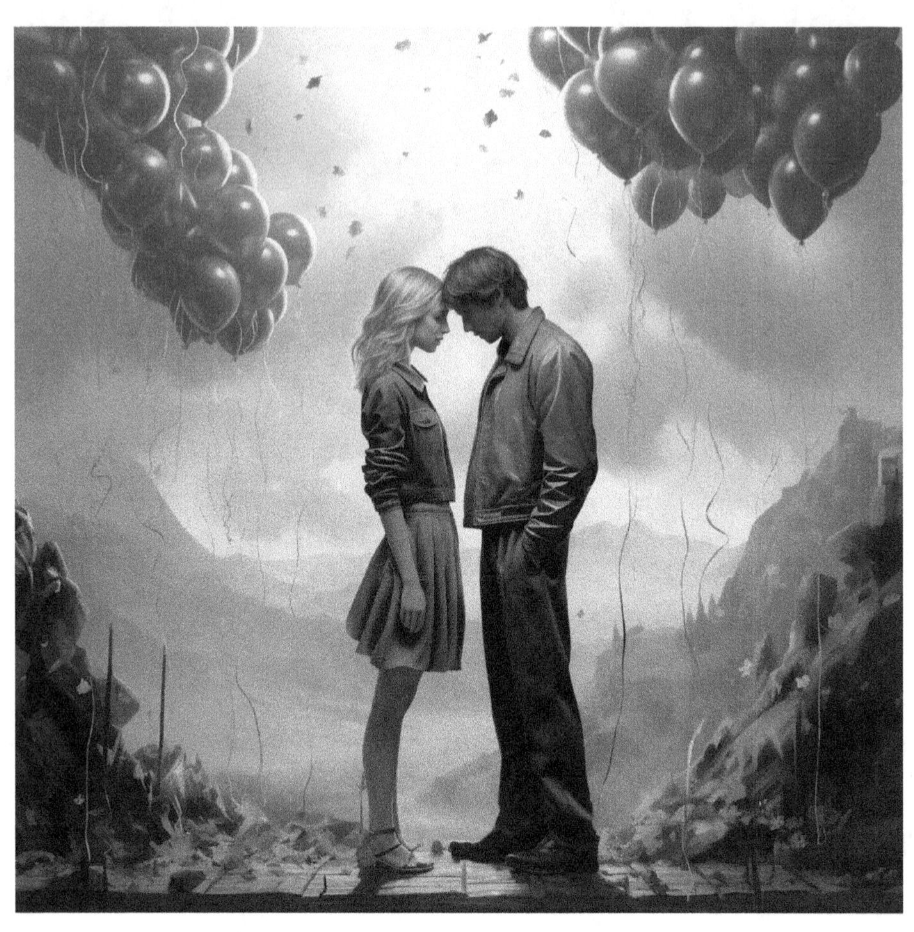

Chapter 4

Figuring It All Out:

Relationships

Welcome to the next chapter of your journey: relationships. In this chapter, we'll explore the complex and fascinating world of romantic connections, friendships, and everything in between. From navigating the highs and lows of dating to cultivating meaningful relationships built on trust and communication, we'll delve into the key ingredients for building strong and fulfilling connections with others.

Relationships are a central aspect of the human experience, shaping our emotions, thoughts, and sense of self. Whether you're embarking on a new romance, nurturing an existing partnership, or navigating the complexities of friendships, understanding the dynamics of relationships is essential for personal growth and fulfillment.

Throughout this chapter, we'll cover a wide range of topics, including communication skills, conflict resolution, building trust, and maintaining healthy boundaries. We'll also explore the different types of relationships, from romantic partnerships to platonic friendships, and discuss strategies for nurturing and sustaining these connections over time.

As you embark on this exploration of relationships, remember that each interaction is an opportunity for growth, learning, and connection. Whether you're seeking love, friendship, or companionship, approach each relationship with an open heart, a curious mind, and a willingness to learn from both the joys and challenges that come your way.

So, let's dive into the world of relationships together and explore the rich tapestry of human connection. Whether you're looking to deepen existing relationships, forge new connections, or simply gain a deeper understanding of the dynamics at play, this chapter is your guide to navigating the intricate web of relationships with grace, compassion, and authenticity.

Types of Relationships: Exploring the Bonds We Form

Relationships come in many shapes and forms, each playing a unique role in shaping our lives and enriching our experiences. In this section, we'll delve into three primary types of relationships: friendships, family connections, and romantic partnerships.

- o **Friendships**: Friends are the family we choose for ourselves, bound together by shared experiences, interests, and mutual support. Friendships can range from casual acquaintances to deep, lifelong bonds, each offering its own blend of companionship, laughter, and emotional support. Whether it's a childhood friend who knows you inside and out or a new acquaintance who brings fresh perspectives and adventures into your life, friendships are an essential part of the human experience.

- o **Family Connections**: Family relationships form the cornerstone of our support systems, providing a sense of belonging, love, and continuity across generations. From parents and siblings to grandparents, aunts, uncles, and cousins, family connections shape our identity and influence our values, beliefs, and behaviors. While family dynamics can be complex and challenging at times, the bonds of family offer a source of strength, comfort, and unconditional love that can withstand the test of time.

- o **Romantic Partnerships**: Romantic relationships are a unique blend of passion, intimacy, and companionship, offering a deep emotional connection and shared journey through life's ups and downs. Whether you're navigating the exhilarating highs of new love or the comforting familiarity of a long-term partnership, romantic relationships provide an opportunity for growth, self-discovery, and mutual support. From romantic gestures and shared adventures to the everyday moments of connection and intimacy, romantic partnerships enrich our lives in profound and meaningful ways.

Each type of relationship brings its own joys, challenges, and opportunities for growth. By nurturing and investing in these connections with care, respect, and authenticity, we can cultivate a rich tapestry of relationships that enrich our lives and bring fulfillment and happiness into our hearts.

In the pages that follow, we'll explore strategies for building and maintaining healthy relationships, fostering open communication, and navigating the complexities of human connection with grace and empathy. Whether you're seeking to strengthen existing relationships or forge new connections, understanding the dynamics of different relationship types is essential for fostering meaningful and fulfilling connections with others.

Friendships: The Family We Choose

Friends are the family we choose for ourselves, forming bonds that are as diverse and dynamic as the individuals who comprise them. From childhood companions to adult confidants, friendships enrich our lives in myriad ways, offering companionship, laughter, and unwavering support through life's joys and challenges.

At the heart of every friendship lies a shared history of experiences, interests, and memories that bind us together. Whether it's bonding over shared hobbies, navigating the complexities of adolescence, or supporting each other through life's milestones, friendships are built on a foundation of mutual understanding and empathy.

Friendships come in all shapes and sizes, ranging from casual acquaintances to deep, lifelong bonds. Some friendships may be fleeting, lasting only for a season, while others endure the test of time, growing stronger with each passing year. Regardless of their duration, each friendship offers a unique blend of companionship, laughter, and emotional support that enriches our lives and enhances our sense of belonging.

Childhood friends hold a special place in our hearts, having witnessed our growth and evolution from a young age. They know us inside and out, sharing in our triumphs and tribulations as we navigate the ups and downs of life together. These lifelong bonds are a testament to the enduring power of friendship, offering a sense of continuity and connection that spans the years.

Yet, friendships are not limited to the past; they are continually evolving and expanding as we journey through life. New acquaintances bring fresh perspectives and adventures into our lives, broadening our horizons and challenging us to grow in new ways. Whether it's a coworker who becomes a trusted confidant or a fellow hobbyist who shares our passion for adventure, these new friendships add depth and richness to our social networks, enriching our lives with diverse experiences and perspectives.

In essence, friendships are an essential part of the human experience, offering companionship, laughter, and emotional support through life's twists and turns. Whether we're laughing together over inside jokes, lending a listening ear during times of need, or simply enjoying each other's company in silence, friendships remind us that we are never alone on this journey called life.

Family Connections: The Bedrock of Support and Love

Family relationships form the bedrock of our support systems, providing a sense of belonging, love, and continuity that transcends time and space. From the earliest days of our lives to the twilight years of old age, family connections shape our identity, influence our values, and profoundly impact the trajectory of our lives.

60

Within the tapestry of family, there are countless threads weaving together the bonds of love and kinship. Parents serve as our first teachers, guiding us with wisdom and nurturing us with unconditional love. Siblings are our partners in mischief, our allies in adventure, and our lifelong confidants. Grandparents offer a wealth of wisdom and experience, sharing stories of the past and imparting lessons for the future. Aunts, uncles, and cousins form the extended branches of our family tree, enriching our lives with laughter, camaraderie, and shared traditions.

While family dynamics can be complex and challenging at times, the bonds of family offer a source of strength, comfort, and unconditional love that can withstand the test of time. Through the highs and lows of life, our family stands by our side, offering unwavering support and a shoulder to lean on when times get tough.

Family connections shape our identity and influence our values, beliefs, and behaviors in profound ways. From the cultural traditions passed down through generations to the shared memories forged in moments of joy and sorrow, our family shapes the lens through which we view the world and the people we become.

Yet, family is not solely defined by blood ties; it is also found in the bonds of chosen family—those individuals who, though not related by blood, become an integral part of our lives through shared experiences and mutual love and respect.

In essence, family connections form the cornerstone of our support systems, providing a sense of belonging, love, and continuity that enriches our lives in immeasurable ways. As we journey through life, let us cherish the bonds of family and celebrate the love and connection that binds us together across generations.

Romantic Partnerships: Navigating the Depths of Connection

Romantic relationships are an intricate dance of passion, intimacy, and companionship, offering a depth of emotional connection that is unlike any other. Whether you're swept up in the whirlwind of new love or reveling in the comfort of a long-term partnership, romantic relationships are a journey of growth, self-discovery, and mutual support.

In the exhilarating throes of new love, every moment feels electrifying as you explore the depths of your connection and discover the intricacies of your partner's soul. From the butterflies in your stomach to the late-night conversations that stretch into the early hours of the morning, new love is a time of excitement, anticipation, and boundless possibility.

Yet, as the relationship matures and deepens, it transforms into a comforting embrace of familiarity and shared experiences. In the quiet moments of everyday life, you find solace in the warmth of your partner's presence and the reassuring rhythm of your shared routines. Together, you weather life's storms and celebrate its triumphs, knowing that you have each other's backs through thick and thin.

Romantic partnerships enrich our lives in profound and meaningful ways, offering a sanctuary of love and acceptance in a world filled with chaos and uncertainty. From grand romantic gestures to the everyday moments of connection and intimacy, each interaction serves to strengthen the bond between partners and deepen their understanding of one another.

In essence, romantic relationships are a journey of discovery and growth, offering an opportunity to explore the depths of connection and intimacy with another soul. Whether you're navigating the exhilarating highs of new love or reveling in the comfort of a long-term partnership, romantic relationships have the power to enrich our lives and fill our hearts with love, joy, and fulfillment.

Romantic relationships stand as a testament to the profound and transformative power of human connection. They are a tapestry woven with threads of passion, intimacy, and companionship, offering a depth of emotional connection that transcends the ordinary and embarks on a shared journey through life's myriad experiences.

In the initial stages of a romantic partnership, the intoxicating rush of new love envelops both individuals in a whirlwind of excitement and possibility. Each moment is tinged with anticipation as they explore the depths of their connection, discovering the nuances of each other's personalities, dreams, and desires. From the stolen glances to the electric touch of hands, every interaction is imbued with a sense of exhilaration and wonder as they navigate the exhilarating highs of infatuation and desire.

As the relationship evolves and matures, it transitions into a comforting haven of familiarity and shared experiences. The initial spark of passion may ebb and flow, but it is replaced by a deeper, more enduring bond built on trust, respect, and mutual understanding. Together, partners weather life's storms and celebrate its triumphs, knowing that they have each other's unwavering support and love to lean on.

Romantic partnerships provide a fertile ground for personal growth and self-discovery, offering individuals the opportunity to confront their fears, insecurities, and vulnerabilities in the presence of a supportive and loving companion. Through the ups and downs of life, partners learn and grow together, forging a stronger, more resilient bond that withstands the test of time.

From grand romantic gestures to the simple pleasures of everyday life, romantic partnerships enrich our lives in profound and meaningful ways. Whether it's embarking on shared adventures, engaging in heartfelt conversations, or simply basking in the warmth of each other's presence, every moment shared with a romantic partner is an opportunity to deepen the bond and nurture the connection that binds two souls together.

Romantic relationships stand as an exquisite fusion of passion, intimacy, and companionship, weaving together the threads of shared experiences and heartfelt connection into a tapestry of love and understanding. They serve as a beacon of light guiding us through life's twists and turns, offering solace, joy, and unwavering support through every triumph and tribulation.

In the exhilarating embrace of new love, every glance, every touch, every whispered word ignites a spark of excitement and possibility. The world seems to shimmer with newfound vibrancy as we explore the depths of our connection with our partner, discovering the unique blend of quirks, dreams, and desires that make them who they are. From the dizzying heights of passion to the tender moments of vulnerability, each interaction is suffused with an electric energy that binds two souls together in a dance of love and desire.

Yet, as the initial fervor of new love gives way to the gentle rhythm of a long-term partnership, a deeper, more profound bond emerges—one rooted in trust, respect, and shared experiences. Together, partners navigate the ebb and flow of life's currents, drawing strength and solace from the unwavering support of their companion. Whether facing challenges or celebrating triumphs, they stand side by side, united in their commitment to each other and to the shared journey they undertake.

Romantic relationships offer a fertile ground for personal growth and self-discovery, providing a mirror through which we can confront our fears, insecurities, and vulnerabilities. In the presence of a loving and supportive partner, we find the courage to peel back the layers of our being, revealing our true selves and embracing our imperfections with grace and acceptance. Through the trials and tribulations of life, we learn and grow together, forging a deeper understanding of ourselves and each other in the process.

From grand romantic gestures to the quiet moments of connection and intimacy, every interaction shared with a romantic partner is an opportunity to deepen the bond and nurture the connection that binds two souls together. Whether embarking on shared adventures, engaging in heartfelt conversations, or simply reveling in the warmth of each other's presence, every moment spent with a beloved partner is a treasure to be cherished and savored.

In essence, romantic partnerships are a celebration of love, connection, and shared humanity—a testament to the transformative power of human connection in all its forms. Whether navigating the exhilarating highs of new love or reveling in the comforting familiarity of a long-term partnership, romantic relationships enrich our lives in profound and meaningful ways, filling our hearts with love, joy, and boundless possibility.

Healthy vs. Unhealthy Relationships: Navigating the Path to Fulfilling Connections

Relationships are the cornerstone of human experience, shaping our emotions, behaviors, and sense of self. Yet, not all relationships are created equal. While healthy relationships are characterized by mutual respect, trust, and open communication, unhealthy relationships may be marked by toxicity, manipulation, and abuse. Understanding the difference between healthy and unhealthy relationships is essential for cultivating fulfilling connections and safeguarding our well-being.

Healthy Relationships:

In healthy relationships, both partners feel valued, respected, and supported. Communication is open, honest, and non-judgmental, allowing each individual to express their thoughts, feelings, and needs freely. Trust forms the foundation of the relationship, with both partners demonstrating reliability, honesty, and integrity in their interactions. Boundaries are established and respected, ensuring that each person's autonomy and individuality are honored.

Healthy relationships are characterized by mutual growth and support, with both partners encouraging and uplifting each other to reach their full potential. Conflict is approached constructively, with a focus on finding solutions and understanding rather than blame or criticism. Partners in healthy relationships celebrate each other's successes, share in each other's joys, and provide comfort and reassurance during times of difficulty.

Unhealthy Relationships:

On the other hand, unhealthy relationships may be characterized by patterns of control, manipulation, and disrespect. One or both partners may feel belittled, invalidated, or diminished in their sense of self-worth. Communication may be characterized by criticism, defensiveness, or stonewalling, leading to misunderstandings and resentment. Trust may be eroded by dishonesty, betrayal, or a lack of transparency in the relationship.

In unhealthy relationships, boundaries may be violated or ignored, leading to feelings of powerlessness and resentment. One partner may exert control over the other through manipulation, coercion, or emotional abuse. Conflict may escalate into arguments or even physical violence, creating a toxic and unsafe environment for both partners.

Navigating the Path:

Recognizing the signs of an unhealthy relationship is the first step toward creating positive change and fostering healthy connections. It's essential to trust your instincts and prioritize your well-being, seeking support from trusted friends, family members, or professionals if needed. Remember that you deserve to be treated with respect, kindness, and dignity in all of your relationships.

By cultivating self-awareness, setting boundaries, and fostering open communication, you can build healthy, fulfilling relationships that bring joy, support, and connection into your life. Whether it's with romantic partners, friends, or family members, investing in healthy relationships is an essential aspect of personal growth and well-being. So, take the time to nurture the connections that uplift and inspire you, and let go of those that no longer serve your highest good.

Breaking Up and Moving On: Navigating the End of Relationships

The end of a relationship can be one of the most challenging experiences we face in life. Whether it's the dissolution of a romantic partnership, the drifting apart of friendships, or the estrangement from family members, the process of letting go and moving on can be fraught with emotions and uncertainties. Yet, it's also an opportunity for growth, self-discovery, and renewed resilience as we navigate the path forward.

Honoring Your Emotions: Allow yourself to feel and process the full range of emotions that come with a breakup—grief, sadness, anger, confusion, and everything in between. It's okay to cry, to vent, to seek support from trusted friends or a therapist, and to give yourself the time and space you need to heal.

Setting Boundaries: Establish clear boundaries with your ex-partner or former friend to protect your emotional well-being and facilitate the healing process. This may involve limiting contact, unfollowing or unfriending them on social media, and refraining from revisiting old memories or shared spaces until you feel ready.

Reflecting on Lessons Learned: Take time to reflect on the relationship and what you've learned from the experience. What were the strengths and weaknesses of the relationship? What patterns or behaviors contributed to its demise? What insights can you carry forward into future relationships to foster healthier connections?

Focusing on Self-Care: Prioritize self-care and nurturing activities that bring you comfort, joy, and fulfillment. Whether it's spending time with loved ones, engaging in hobbies and interests, practicing mindfulness and meditation, or seeking professional support, prioritize activities that nourish your body, mind, and spirit.

Embracing New Beginnings: While the end of a relationship may feel like the end of the road, it's also an opportunity for new beginnings and fresh starts. Embrace the journey of self-discovery and personal growth that comes with moving on from the past, and open yourself up to new experiences, connections, and possibilities.

Seeking Closure: Closure is a deeply personal process that looks different for everyone. It may involve having a conversation with your ex-partner or friend to gain clarity and closure, writing a letter that you never intend to send, or simply finding closure within yourself through self-reflection and acceptance.

Staying Optimistic: Remember that healing takes time, and it's okay to have setbacks along the way. Stay patient, kind, and compassionate with yourself as you navigate the ups and downs of the healing journey. Trust that brighter days are ahead and that you have the strength and resilience to overcome any challenge that comes your way.

Breaking up and moving on from a relationship is never easy, but it's also an opportunity for growth, healing, and transformation. By honoring your emotions, setting boundaries, reflecting on lessons learned, prioritizing self-care, embracing new beginnings, seeking closure, and staying optimistic, you can navigate the end of a relationship with grace, resilience, and self-compassion. Remember that you are not alone in this journey, and that with time and support, you will emerge stronger, wiser, and more resilient than ever before.

As we come to the end of this chapter on breaking up and moving on, it's important to acknowledge the strength and courage it takes to navigate the complexities of ending a relationship. Whether you're grappling with the end of a romantic partnership, the drifting apart of friendships, or the estrangement from family members, the process of letting go and moving forward can be incredibly challenging.

But it's also a journey of growth, self-discovery, and resilience—a testament to the power of the human spirit to overcome adversity and emerge stronger on the other side. By honoring your emotions, setting boundaries, seeking support, and embracing the opportunities for growth and renewal that come with letting go, you can navigate the end of a relationship with grace, courage, and self-compassion.

Remember that healing takes time, and it's okay to take things one day at a time. Trust in your inner strength and resilience, and know that brighter days lie ahead. As you continue on your journey of healing and self-discovery, may you find solace in the knowledge that you are not alone, and that with time, support, and self-compassion, you will emerge from this experience stronger, wiser, and more empowered than ever before.

So take a deep breath, trust in the process, and know that you are capable of overcoming any challenge that comes your way. The road ahead may be uncertain, but it's also filled with infinite possibilities for growth, happiness, and fulfillment. Embrace the journey with an open heart and a resilient spirit, and know that you have everything you need to create a life that is full of love, joy, and meaning.

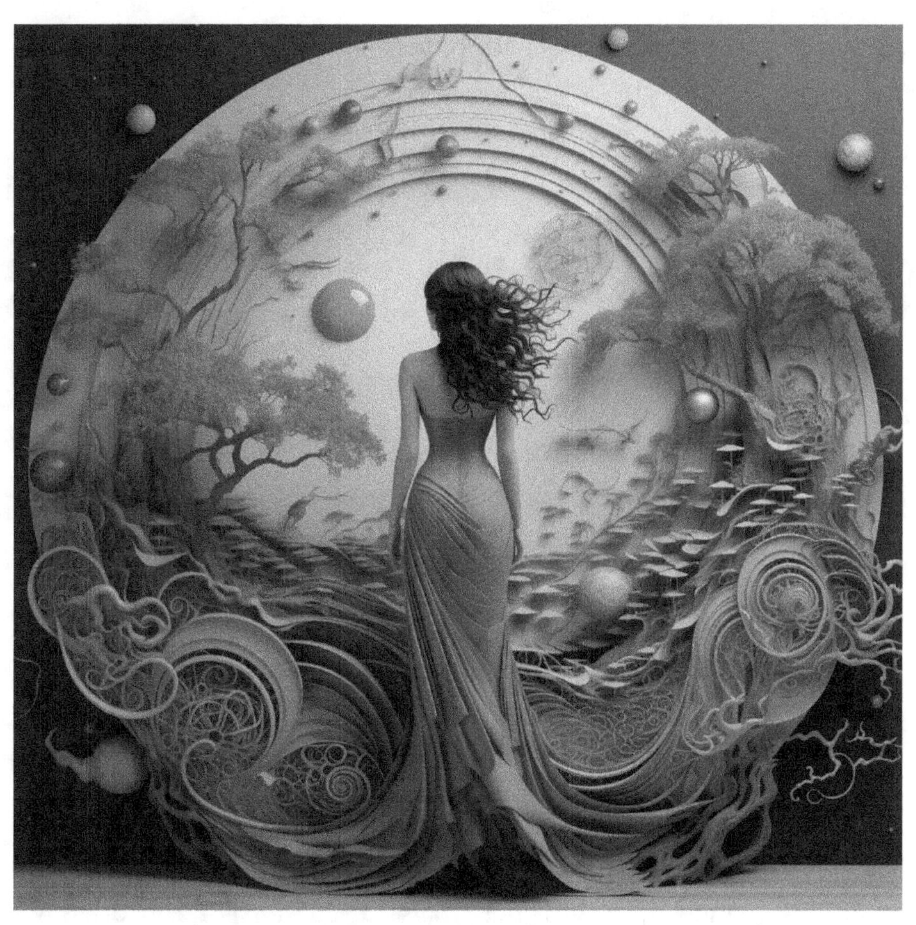

Chapter 5

Understanding the Menstrual Cycle

Before delving into the intricacies of the menstrual cycle, it's essential to lay the groundwork by understanding the fundamental differences in anatomy between individuals assigned female at birth (AFAB) and those assigned male at birth (AMAB). While both sexes share many similarities in their reproductive organs, there are distinct physiological differences that shape their experiences of puberty, fertility, and reproductive health.

Differences in Anatomy: Exploring the Biological Variances

Individuals assigned female at birth possess reproductive anatomy that includes structures such as the ovaries, fallopian tubes, uterus, and vagina. The ovaries are responsible for producing eggs (ova) and releasing hormones such as estrogen and progesterone, which regulate the menstrual cycle and support pregnancy. The fallopian tubes serve as conduits for the transport of eggs from the ovaries to the uterus, where fertilization may occur. The uterus, also known as the womb, is the site of embryo implantation and fetal development during pregnancy. The vagina serves as a passageway for menstrual blood, sexual intercourse, and childbirth.

In contrast, individuals assigned male at birth have reproductive anatomy that includes structures such as the testes, vas deferens, seminal vesicles, prostate gland, and penis. The testes are responsible for producing sperm and secreting hormones such as testosterone, which play a key role in the development of secondary sexual characteristics and the maintenance of reproductive function. The vas deferens carries sperm from the testes to the urethra, where it is ejaculated during sexual intercourse. The seminal vesicles and prostate gland produce seminal fluid, which nourishes and protects sperm during ejaculation. The penis serves as the external organ of the male reproductive system, facilitating sexual intercourse and the delivery of sperm into the female reproductive tract.

Understanding Puberty and Hormonal Changes

Puberty marks the transition from childhood to adulthood and is characterized by significant hormonal changes and physical development. In individuals assigned female at birth, puberty typically begins between the ages of 8 and 13 and is initiated by the release of hormones such as estrogen and progesterone from the ovaries. This hormonal surge triggers the development of secondary sexual characteristics such as breast development, pubic hair growth, and the onset of menstruation.

In individuals assigned male at birth, puberty typically begins between the ages of 9 and 14 and is initiated by the release of hormones such as testosterone from the testes. This hormonal surge triggers the development of secondary sexual characteristics such as facial hair growth, deepening of the voice, and enlargement of the Adam's apple.

By understanding the basic differences in anatomy and the hormonal changes that occur during puberty, individuals can gain insight into the unique experiences of AFAB and AMAB individuals and the reproductive health challenges they may face. With this foundation in place, we can now explore the menstrual cycle in more detail, delving into its phases, hormonal fluctuations, and the physical and emotional changes that accompany each stage. Through knowledge and understanding, we can empower individuals to take control of their reproductive health and well-being.

The Menstrual Cycle: Your Body's Monthly Adventure

Okay, let's talk about something that might seem mysterious but is actually totally normal: your menstrual cycle. This is the monthly journey your body takes, and it's all about getting ready for the possibility of making a baby.

The Basics: What Happens Each Month

So, here's the deal: Every month, your body gets ready for the possibility of pregnancy. It's like your body saying, "Hey, let's get ready, just in case!" Here's how it goes down:

1. **Getting Started**: First off, your uterus (that's the place where a baby grows if you get pregnant) starts building up its lining with blood and tissue. This is just in case an egg gets fertilized by sperm and needs a cozy place to grow.

2. **Egg Time**: Around the middle of your cycle (that's about two weeks before your period starts), your ovary releases an egg. This is called ovulation. If the egg meets up with sperm, it can turn into a baby.

3. **Waiting Game**: If the egg doesn't meet up with any sperm, your body says, "Okay, guess we don't need this extra stuff," and it gets rid of the lining it built up. That's when you get your period.

4. **Back to Square One**: After your period ends, your body starts the whole process over again. It's like hitting the reset button on your menstrual cycle.

What You Might Notice

Your menstrual cycle isn't just about what's happening inside your body; it can also affect how you feel and what you notice happening on the outside. Here are some things you might notice:

- **Period Pals**: When your period shows up, you might notice some bleeding. It can be light or heavy, and it might last a few days or up to a week.

- **Crampy Vibes**: Some people get cramps during their period. These can feel like a dull ache or a sharp pain in your belly.

- **Mood Swings**: Your hormones can do some funky stuff during your cycle, which might make you feel moody or emotional. It's totally normal to feel like you're on an emotional rollercoaster sometimes.

- **Pimples and Bloated Belly**: Hormones can also mess with your skin and make you feel bloated or puffy.

Taking Care of You

Dealing with your period might seem like a hassle sometimes, but it's all part of being a healthy, normal person. Here are some things you can do to take care of yourself during your menstrual cycle:

- **Stay Comfortable**: If you're feeling crampy or bloated, try using a heating pad or taking a warm bath to help you feel better.

- **Be Prepared**: Keep some pads, tampons, or menstrual cups handy so you're ready when your period shows up.

- o **Talk About It:** If you're feeling confused or worried about your period, don't be shy about talking to a trusted adult or healthcare provider. They can help answer your questions and make sure everything's okay.

- o **Listen to Your Body**: Pay attention to how you feel during your menstrual cycle. If something doesn't seem right or if you're having really bad symptoms, talk to someone about it.

Remember, your menstrual cycle is a totally normal part of being a person with a uterus, and there's nothing to be ashamed or embarrassed about. So embrace your body, take care of yourself, and know that you're not alone on this monthly adventure!

Understanding the Menstrual Cycle: Navigating the Rhythms of Womanhood

The menstrual cycle is a natural and intricate process that occurs in the bodies of people with ovaries, typically lasting around 28 days, although it can vary from person to person. This chapter aims to shed light on the various phases of the menstrual cycle, the hormones involved, and the physical and emotional changes that accompany each stage. By gaining a deeper understanding of the menstrual cycle, individuals can better manage their reproductive health and well-being.

1. **Menstrual Phase**: The menstrual phase marks the beginning of the menstrual cycle and is characterized by the shedding of the uterine lining, resulting in menstrual bleeding. This phase typically lasts around 3 to 7 days and is influenced by fluctuations in hormone levels, particularly estrogen and progesterone. While menstrual bleeding can be accompanied by physical symptoms such as cramps, fatigue, and headaches, it is a normal and natural part of the menstrual cycle.

2. **Follicular Phase**: Following the menstrual phase, the follicular phase begins, lasting approximately 7 to 10 days. During this phase, hormone levels begin to rise, stimulating the development of ovarian follicles in preparation for ovulation. Estrogen levels increase, causing the uterine lining to thicken in anticipation of a potential pregnancy. Additionally, cervical mucus becomes thinner and more watery, creating a hospitable environment for sperm to travel through the reproductive tract.

3. **Ovulation**: Ovulation marks the midpoint of the menstrual cycle and occurs around day 14 in a typical 28-day cycle. During ovulation, a mature egg is released from one of the ovarian follicles and travels down the fallopian tube, where it may be fertilized by sperm. Ovulation is triggered by a surge in luteinizing hormone (LH), which causes the ovarian follicle to rupture and release the egg. This phase is characterized by increased cervical mucus production and a slight rise in basal body temperature.

4. **Luteal Phase**: Following ovulation, the luteal phase begins, lasting approximately 10 to 14 days. During this phase, the ruptured ovarian follicle transforms into a structure called the corpus luteum, which produces progesterone to support the thickened uterine lining. If fertilization does not occur, hormone levels decline, leading to the shedding of the uterine lining and the onset of menstruation. The luteal phase is characterized by hormonal fluctuations that can impact mood, energy levels, and physical symptoms such as breast tenderness and bloating.

By understanding the menstrual cycle and the various phases it encompasses, individuals can gain insight into their reproductive health and well-being. Tracking menstrual cycles can also help identify patterns and irregularities that may warrant further investigation by a healthcare provider. Ultimately, by fostering a deeper understanding of the menstrual cycle, individuals can take proactive steps to manage their reproductive health and empower themselves to make informed decisions about their bodies and their lives.

Hormonal Changes and Their Effects: The Symphony of Reproductive Hormones

The menstrual cycle is intricately regulated by a delicate interplay of hormones, each playing a vital role in orchestrating the various physiological changes that occur throughout its duration. Understanding the fluctuations in hormonal levels and their effects on the body is essential for comprehending the menstrual cycle and managing reproductive health effectively.

1. **Estrogen**: Estrogen is often referred to as the "female" hormone, although it is present in both AFAB and AMAB individuals. Produced primarily by the ovaries, estrogen plays a key role in regulating the menstrual cycle and supporting reproductive function. During the follicular phase of the menstrual cycle, estrogen levels rise, stimulating the thickening of the uterine lining in preparation for potential pregnancy. Estrogen also influences secondary sexual characteristics such as breast development, fat distribution, and bone density.

2. **Progesterone**: Progesterone is another crucial hormone involved in the menstrual cycle, primarily produced by the ovaries following ovulation. During the luteal phase of the menstrual cycle, progesterone levels rise, maintaining the thickened uterine lining and preparing the body for implantation of a fertilized egg. If fertilization does not occur, progesterone levels decline, triggering the shedding of the uterine lining and the onset of menstruation.

78

3. **Luteinizing Hormone (LH):** Luteinizing hormone is produced by the pituitary gland and plays a key role in triggering ovulation. A surge in LH levels occurs around day 14 of the menstrual cycle, causing the dominant ovarian follicle to rupture and release a mature egg from the ovary. This surge in LH is essential for the timing of ovulation and the release of the egg into the fallopian tube, where it may be fertilized by sperm.

4. **Follicle-Stimulating Hormone (FSH):** Follicle-stimulating hormone is also produced by the pituitary gland and plays a crucial role in the development of ovarian follicles. FSH stimulates the growth and maturation of ovarian follicles in the ovaries during the follicular phase of the menstrual cycle, preparing them for ovulation. Elevated levels of FSH are essential for the recruitment and selection of a dominant follicle that will ovulate during the menstrual cycle.

5. **Testosterone:** Although often associated with male reproductive health, testosterone is also present in AFAB individuals and plays a role in regulating the menstrual cycle. Testosterone is produced by the ovaries and adrenal glands and influences libido, energy levels, and muscle mass. While testosterone levels are lower in AFAB individuals compared to AMAB individuals, they still contribute to overall reproductive health and well-being.

Effects of Hormonal Fluctuations

Fluctuations in hormonal levels throughout the menstrual cycle can have a wide range of effects on the body, influencing physical, emotional, and cognitive functioning. These effects may include:

o Changes in menstrual bleeding patterns, including the length and intensity of menstruation.

- o Physical symptoms such as breast tenderness, bloating, acne, and headaches.

- o Emotional symptoms such as mood swings, irritability, anxiety, and depression.

- o Changes in libido and sexual arousal.

- o Cognitive changes such as difficulty concentrating, memory lapses, and changes in appetite.

By understanding the hormonal changes that occur during the menstrual cycle and their effects on the body, individuals can gain insight into their reproductive health and well-being. Tracking menstrual cycles and monitoring symptoms can help identify patterns and irregularities that may warrant further investigation by a healthcare provider. Ultimately, by fostering a deeper understanding of hormonal fluctuations, individuals can take proactive steps to manage their reproductive health effectively and navigate the menstrual cycle with confidence and grace.

As we wrap up this chapter on the menstrual cycle, it's important to remember that your body is amazing and capable of incredible things. Your menstrual cycle might seem like a hassle sometimes, but it's actually a sign that your body is healthy and doing what it's supposed to do.

So, whether you're in the middle of your period, gearing up for ovulation, or just taking a break in between cycles, take a moment to appreciate your body and all the incredible things it does for you.

Your menstrual cycle is just one part of what makes you unique, and it's nothing to be ashamed of or embarrassed about. So embrace your body, embrace your cycle, and know that you're not alone on this journey. Reach out to friends, family, or healthcare providers if you have questions or concerns, and remember that there's a whole community of people out there who are going through the same thing as you.

As you continue on your journey of self-discovery and growth, may you find strength, resilience, and empowerment in the knowledge that you are beautifully and wonderfully made, just as you are. Here's to embracing your body, embracing your cycle, and embracing yourself, exactly as you are. You've got this!

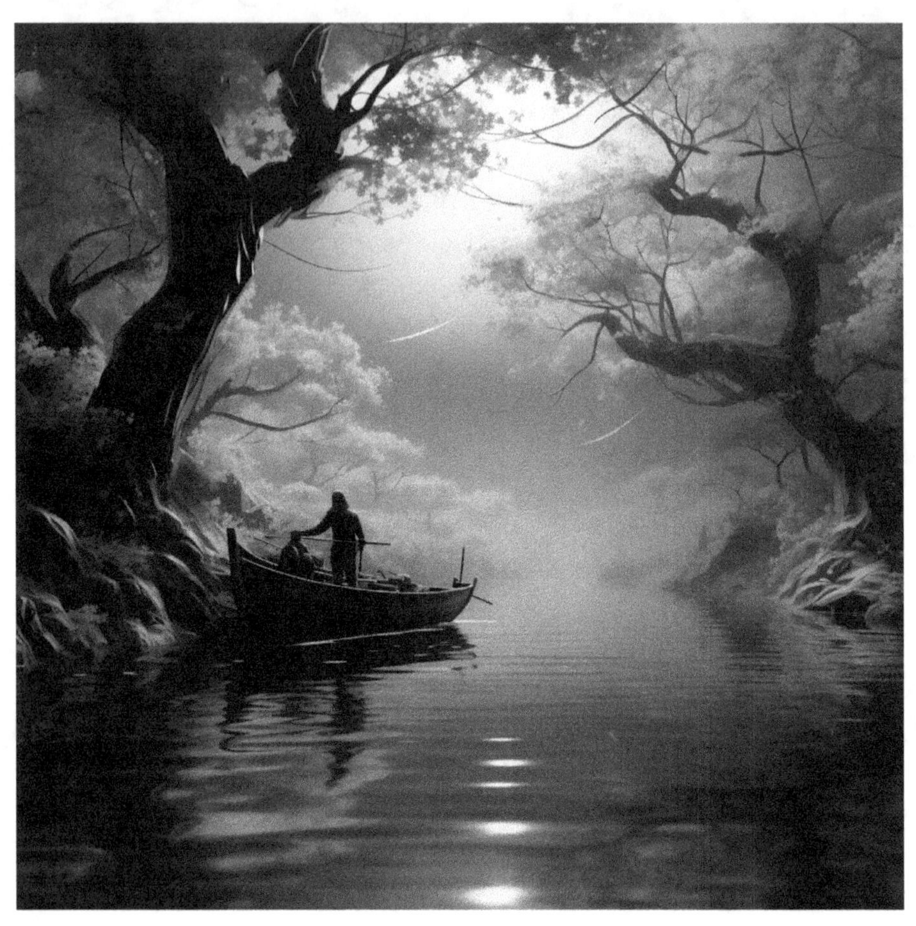

Chapter 6

Navigating Sexual Feelings

Sexual feelings can be a bit like a rollercoaster ride—exciting, thrilling, and sometimes a little scary. But don't worry, you're not alone in experiencing them. As you journey through your teenage years, you might start noticing new sensations, thoughts, and desires cropping up, and that's all completely normal.

So, what are sexual feelings, exactly? Well, they're a natural part of being human. Your body is wired to feel pleasure and desire, and those feelings can manifest in a variety of ways. It might be a fluttery feeling in your stomach when you're around someone you're attracted to, a rush of excitement when you think about kissing or touching, or even just a general curiosity about sex and relationships.

But here's the thing: sexual feelings can be pretty complex, and they can mean different things to different people. Some folks might start feeling curious about sex at a younger age, while others might not feel those feelings until they're older. Some might feel attracted to people of the same gender, opposite gender, or multiple genders, while others might not feel much attraction at all.

And that's all okay! There's no right or wrong way to feel, and there's certainly no rush to figure it all out. Your sexual feelings are yours to explore and understand at your own pace, and it's important to give yourself the time and space to do so without judgment or pressure.

Of course, navigating sexual feelings can sometimes feel a bit overwhelming or confusing, especially if you're not sure what to make of them. You might have questions like:

- What do these feelings mean?

- Is it normal to feel this way?

- How do I know if I'm ready for sex or a relationship?

- What if I'm attracted to someone but they're not attracted to me?

- How do I stay safe and make responsible choices?

These are all valid questions, and it's okay to seek out answers and support as you navigate your sexual journey. Talking to trusted adults, friends, or healthcare providers can be a great way to get the information and guidance you need to feel more confident and empowered in your choices.

Remember, your sexual feelings are a natural and normal part of growing up, and there's no shame in exploring them and seeking out the knowledge and support you need along the way. So embrace your curiosity, honor your desires, and know that you're not alone on this journey. You've got this!

Sexual attraction is like a mysterious force that can pull you towards someone in a way that's hard to explain. It's that feeling you get when you see someone who just seems to light up the room, and you can't help but feel drawn to them.

But what exactly is sexual attraction, and why does it happen? Well, let's break it down a bit.

At its core, sexual attraction is a combination of physical, emotional, and even intellectual factors that make you feel drawn to someone in a romantic or sexual way. It's like a spark that ignites between two people, creating a sense of chemistry and connection that can be incredibly powerful.

Physical attraction is often the first thing that comes to mind when we think about sexual attraction. It's that immediate, gut-level reaction you have when you see someone who just seems to "click" with you on a physical level. Maybe it's their smile, their eyes, or just the way they carry themselves. Whatever it is, there's something about them that makes your heart race and your palms sweat.

But sexual attraction isn't just about looks. It's also about personality, energy, and vibe. You might feel attracted to someone because of their sense of humor, their intelligence, or the way they make you feel when you're around them. It's like there's a magnetic pull between you that's hard to resist.

Of course, sexual attraction can be complicated, and it doesn't always happen in a straightforward way. You might find yourself feeling attracted to someone one day and then not feeling it the next. Or you might feel attracted to someone who doesn't feel the same way about you, which can be tough to navigate.

But here's the thing: sexual attraction is totally normal and natural, and there's no right or wrong way to experience it. It's all about finding what feels right for you and honoring your own feelings and desires.

So if you find yourself feeling attracted to someone, don't be afraid to explore those feelings and see where they lead. Just remember to communicate openly and honestly, respect boundaries, and prioritize your own well-being and comfort. And if things don't work out the way you hoped, that's okay too. There are plenty of other fish in the sea, and you never know what—or who—might come along next.

Alright, let's dive deeper into understanding sexual attraction. It's this incredible force that can leave you feeling butterflies in your stomach and make your heart skip a beat. But what exactly is it and how does it work?

Sexual attraction is like a mysterious dance between you and someone else. It's a combination of physical, emotional, and even intellectual factors that draw you to another person in a romantic or sexual way. Here's a breakdown of what might be going on:

1. **Physical Attraction**: This is usually the first thing that grabs your attention. It's that magnetic pull you feel when you see someone who just seems to have that special something. Maybe it's their smile, their eyes, or their body language—it's different for everyone. Physical attraction is all about those initial sparks that fly when you're around someone who catches your eye.

2. **Emotional Connection**: Beyond the physical stuff, there's also the emotional side of attraction. It's about how you feel when you're with someone, the way they make you laugh, or the deep conversations you have together. Emotional attraction is about forming a bond with someone that goes beyond the surface and makes you feel understood and valued.

3. **Chemistry and Compatibility**: Ever meet someone and just instantly click? That's chemistry at work. It's that special connection you feel with someone that makes everything just feel right. Compatibility is about being on the same wavelength as someone else, sharing similar interests, values, and goals. When you have chemistry and compatibility with someone, it can feel like you've found your perfect match.

Navigating the Waters

Understanding sexual attraction is one thing, but navigating it can be a whole other ballgame. It's important to remember that attraction is a natural and normal part of being human, and there's no right or wrong way to experience it.

If you find yourself feeling attracted to someone, that's totally okay! It's a natural response to finding someone who resonates with you on a deeper level. Just remember to communicate openly and respectfully, respect boundaries, and prioritize your own well-being and comfort.

On the flip side, if someone is attracted to you and you don't feel the same way, that's okay too. It's important to be honest and upfront with them while still being kind and compassionate. Remember, you're not obligated to reciprocate someone's feelings just because they like you.

Ultimately, understanding sexual attraction is about tuning into your own feelings and desires, being true to yourself, and treating others with kindness and respect. So embrace your attractions, explore your connections, and remember that the journey of love and attraction is a beautiful and exciting adventure.

The Layers of Attraction: Delving Deeper into Sexual Attraction

Let's peel back the layers of sexual attraction and explore what makes it tick. Attraction isn't just about physical appearance or chemistry—it's a multi-dimensional experience that involves your mind, body, and soul.

1. **Physical Magnetism**: Physical attraction is often what catches our attention first. It's that instant spark you feel when you see someone who makes your heart skip a beat. Maybe it's their smile, their eyes, or the way they move—it's different for everyone. Physical attraction is like a magnet pulling you towards someone, and it can be electrifying.

2. **Emotional Connection**: Beyond the surface level, there's the emotional aspect of attraction. It's about how someone makes you feel when you're with them—their warmth, their humor, their kindness. Emotional attraction is about forming a deep connection with someone that goes beyond the physical. It's feeling understood, supported, and valued in their presence.

3. **Shared Values and Goals**: Compatibility plays a crucial role in attraction too. It's about finding someone who shares your interests, values, and aspirations. When you meet someone who aligns with your beliefs and dreams, it creates a sense of harmony and connection. Shared values can be a powerful bonding force that strengthens your attraction to someone.

4. **Intellectual Stimulation**: Ever have a conversation that leaves you feeling intellectually stimulated and energized? That's intellectual attraction at work. It's about connecting with someone on an intellectual level, sharing ideas, and

engaging in stimulating conversations. Intellectual attraction can deepen your connection with someone and add another layer of attraction to the mix.

5. **Spiritual Alignment**: For some people, spiritual compatibility is an essential aspect of attraction. It's about sharing a sense of purpose, spirituality, or worldview with someone else. When you feel spiritually aligned with someone, it creates a profound sense of connection and understanding that goes beyond the physical realm.

Cultural Influences and Societal Norms: It's essential to recognize that our perceptions of sexual attraction can also be shaped by cultural influences and societal norms. What we find attractive or desirable can be influenced by the media, advertising, and the people around us. Society often portrays certain traits or characteristics as more attractive or desirable than others, which can impact how we view ourselves and others.

For example, mainstream media often promotes narrow standards of beauty and attractiveness that may not reflect the diversity of human experiences and preferences. This can lead to feelings of insecurity or inadequacy if we don't fit into these narrow standards.

Additionally, societal norms and expectations around gender roles and relationships can influence how we express and experience sexual attraction. These norms may dictate who we're "supposed" to be attracted to, how we're supposed to express our desires, and what types of relationships are considered acceptable.

It's essential to critically examine these cultural influences and question whether they align with our own values, beliefs, and desires. By challenging societal norms and embracing diversity in attraction and expression, we can create more inclusive and affirming spaces for everyone to explore their sexual feelings and identities.

Understanding sexual attraction means recognizing that it's a complex interplay of various factors, each contributing to the overall experience. It's about tuning into your instincts, listening to your heart, and being open to the magic of connection. So embrace the layers of attraction, explore what draws you to others, and remember that attraction is a beautiful, multifaceted phenomenon that enriches our lives in countless ways.

Masturbation and Sexual Exploration: Getting to Know Your Body

Masturbation and sexual exploration are natural and healthy aspects of human sexuality. They're ways for you to learn about your body, discover what feels good, and explore your desires in a safe and private way.

1. What is Masturbation?

Masturbation is when you touch yourself in a way that feels good sexually. It can involve stimulating your genitals with your hands or using objects like vibrators. Masturbation isn't just about reaching orgasm—it's about exploring your body and experiencing pleasure.

2. Why Do People Masturbate?

People masturbate for many reasons. It can be a way to relieve stress, release sexual tension, or simply because it feels good. Masturbation can also help you learn about your body's responses to touch and stimulation, which can be valuable information for sexual activities with a partner.

3. Is Masturbation Normal?

Yes, masturbation is entirely normal and healthy. It's a common behavior that people of all genders and ages engage in.

Masturbation doesn't harm your body or your health—in fact, it can have several benefits, including reducing stress, improving mood, and promoting better sleep.

4. Exploring Your Sexual Fantasies

Fantasies are a natural part of human sexuality. They're the images, thoughts, or scenarios that turn you on and arouse you sexually. Fantasies can range from simple daydreams to elaborate scenarios, and they're entirely normal and healthy.

5. Exploring Different Techniques

There's no right or wrong way to masturbate—it's all about what feels good for you. Experiment with different techniques, speeds, pressures, and rhythms to see what you enjoy the most. You can also explore different erogenous zones on your body, like your nipples, inner thighs, or neck, to see what sensations they produce.

6. Communication and Consent

If you're in a sexual relationship, it's essential to communicate openly and honestly with your partner about your desires, boundaries, and preferences. Consent is crucial in any sexual encounter, including masturbation. Make sure you have your partner's consent before incorporating masturbation into your sexual activities together.

7. Privacy and Safety

Privacy is essential when it comes to masturbation. Find a private space where you feel comfortable and won't be interrupted. It's also essential to practice good hygiene by washing your hands before and after masturbating and cleaning any sex toys you use.

8. Embracing Pleasure

Ultimately, masturbation and sexual exploration are about embracing pleasure and enjoying your body. It's a way to connect with yourself on a deep and intimate level and to celebrate the joy of sexuality. So go ahead, explore your desires, and remember that your body is beautiful, and your pleasure matters.

Understanding Sexual Orientation and Gender Identity

Sexual orientation and gender identity are important aspects of who we are as individuals. Let's dive into what these terms mean and how they can shape our experiences of sexuality and identity.

1. Sexual Orientation:

Sexual orientation refers to who you're attracted to romantically, emotionally, and sexually. It's about the gender(s) of the people you're drawn to and feel connected with. Here are some common sexual orientations:

- **Heterosexual**: Someone who's attracted to people of a different gender.

- **Homosexual**: Someone who's attracted to people of the same gender.

- **Bisexual**: Someone who's attracted to people of more than one gender.

- **Pansexual**: Someone who's attracted to people regardless of their gender.

- **Asexual**: Someone who experiences little or no sexual attraction to others.

Remember, sexual orientation is fluid and can change over time. It's also okay if you're not sure which label fits you best—what matters most is how you feel and who you're attracted to.

2. Gender Identity:

Gender identity is how you personally understand and experience your own gender. It's about whether you identify as male, female, a blend of both, or neither. Some common gender identities include:

- o **Cisgender**: Someone whose gender identity aligns with the sex they were assigned at birth.

- o **Transgender**: Someone whose gender identity differs from the sex they were assigned at birth.

- o **Non-binary**: Someone who identifies as neither strictly male nor strictly female, or as a combination of both.

- o **Genderqueer**: Someone whose gender identity falls outside the traditional binary of male and female.

- o **Genderfluid**: Someone whose gender identity shifts or changes over time.

Gender identity is deeply personal and may not always align with societal expectations or norms. It's important to respect and affirm each person's gender identity, regardless of whether it matches our own understanding or beliefs.

3. Exploring Your Identity:

Exploring your sexual orientation and gender identity can be a journey of self-discovery and self-acceptance. It's okay to take your time and explore different aspects of your identity until you find what feels right for you.

Remember, there's no right or wrong way to be, and it's okay to be yourself. Surround yourself with supportive and accepting people who respect and affirm your identity, and know that you're not alone on this journey. Embrace who you are, celebrate your uniqueness, and know that you are valid and worthy just as you are.

In this chapter, we explored the intricate landscape of sexual feelings and identities, covering a range of topics relevant to teens navigating their sexuality. We began by discussing the importance of understanding oneself, including exploring identity, embracing body positivity and self-love, and addressing emotions and mental health.

Moving forward, we delved into the realm of interpersonal connections, touching on friendships, family relationships, and romantic partnerships. We emphasized the significance of healthy communication, mutual respect, and consent in fostering fulfilling and respectful relationships.

Additionally, we shed light on the menstrual cycle, offering insights into its biological processes, hormonal changes, and practical tips for managing menstrual health and hygiene.

Further, we navigated the complexities of sexual attraction, dissecting its various dimensions and discussing its influences, including biological, psychological, cultural, and societal factors.

We encouraged teens to explore their desires with openness, curiosity, and respect for themselves and others.

Finally, we addressed the diverse aspects of sexual orientation and gender identity, recognizing the fluidity and complexity of human experiences. We emphasized the importance of self-acceptance, affirmation, and support in embracing one's identity and respecting the identities of others.

Throughout this chapter, our aim has been to provide teens with the knowledge, understanding, and empowerment to navigate their sexual feelings and identities with confidence, respect, and authenticity. By fostering open dialogue, self-awareness, and acceptance, we hope to support teens on their journey of sexual exploration and self-discovery.

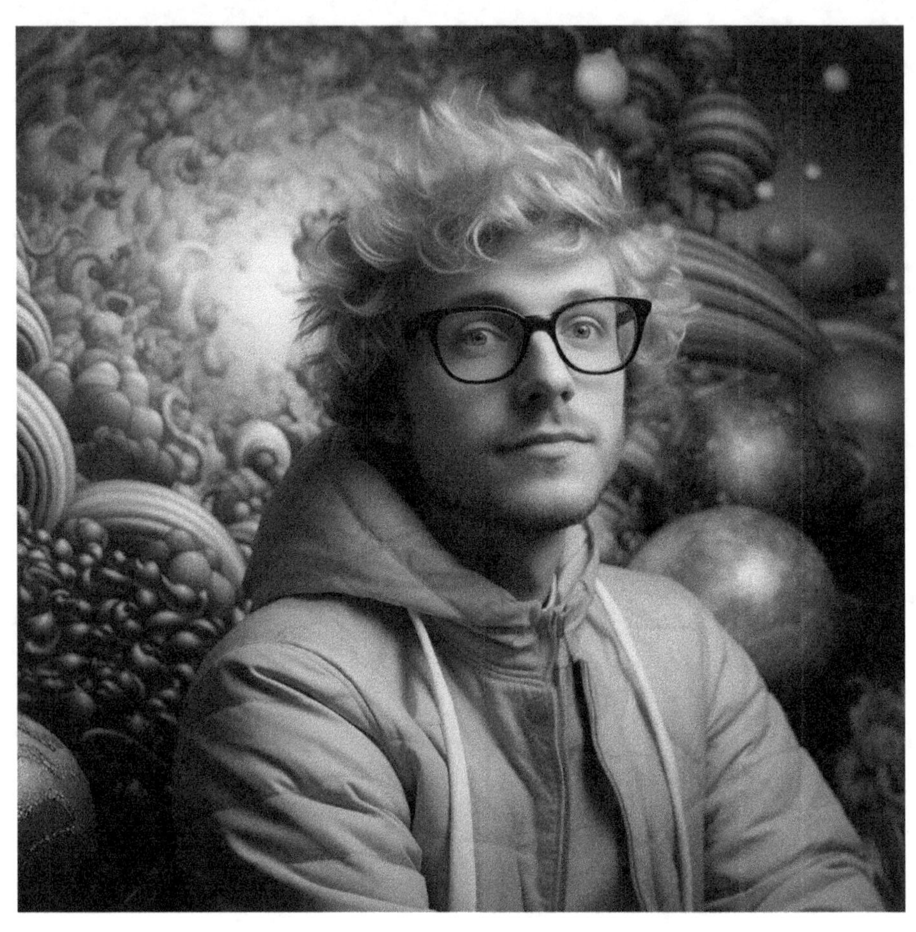

Chapter 7

Safe Sex and Sexual Health

Welcome to the chapter on safe sex and sexual health! In this section, we'll delve into essential information about protecting yourself and your partner(s) while exploring your sexuality. Let's start by understanding the importance of safe sex practices and maintaining sexual health.

Understanding Safe Sex:

Safe sex refers to practices that reduce the risk of sexually transmitted infections (STIs) and unintended pregnancies. It's about taking proactive steps to protect yourself and your partner(s) during sexual activities.

1. Condom Use:

Condoms are one of the most effective tools for preventing STIs and pregnancy. They create a barrier that prevents bodily fluids from being exchanged during sex. Whether you're having vaginal, anal, or oral sex, using condoms consistently and correctly can significantly reduce the risk of transmission.

2. Birth Control:

If you're engaging in vaginal intercourse and don't want to get pregnant, using a form of birth control is essential. There are many options available, including hormonal methods like the pill, patch, or contraceptive injection, as well as non-hormonal methods like the copper IUD or condoms.

3. Communication:

Open and honest communication with your partner(s) is crucial for practicing safe sex. Talk about your sexual history, STI testing, and contraceptive preferences before engaging in sexual activities. Establishing boundaries, consent, and mutual respect is essential for a healthy and enjoyable sexual experience.

4. STI Testing:

Getting tested for STIs regularly is an important part of sexual health maintenance, especially if you have multiple partners or engage in high-risk behaviors. Many STIs don't show symptoms, so getting tested regularly ensures early detection and treatment if necessary.

5. Consent:

Consent is the cornerstone of healthy and respectful sexual interactions. It means that all parties involved willingly agree to engage in sexual activities without coercion or pressure. Remember, consent must be enthusiastic, ongoing, and freely given by all parties involved.

6. Safer Sex Practices:

In addition to condom use and birth control, there are other safer sex practices you can incorporate into your sexual activities. These include avoiding sharing needles or injecting equipment, using dental dams or condoms for oral sex, and reducing alcohol or drug use during sexual encounters.

By prioritizing safe sex practices and maintaining open communication with your partner(s), you can enjoy a fulfilling and healthy sexual life while minimizing the risks of STIs and unintended pregnancies. In the next sections, we'll dive deeper into specific aspects of sexual health, including STI prevention, contraception, and sexual wellness. Stay tuned!

Condom Use: Protecting Your Health

Condoms are like superheroes in the world of safe sex—they're here to protect you from STIs and unplanned pregnancies. Let's talk about why they're so awesome and how to use them like a pro.

Why Condoms Rock:

First off, condoms are super effective at preventing the spread of sexually transmitted infections (STIs) and stopping those little swimmers from reaching their destination and causing a surprise pregnancy. They work by creating a barrier that stops bodily fluids, like semen and vaginal fluids, from mixing during sex. This means that whether you're having vaginal, anal, or oral sex, using condoms consistently and correctly can seriously lower the chances of passing on or catching an STI or getting pregnant.

Using Condoms Correctly:

Now, here's the important part—how to use condoms the right way. First, check the expiration date to make sure your condom is still good to go. Then, carefully open the packet without using your teeth or scissors, as you don't want to accidentally tear the condom. Next, make sure the condom is the right way round—there's usually a little tip that should be facing upwards. Pinch the tip to leave some space for semen, then roll the condom down the shaft of the penis or onto whatever object you're using for penetration. After sex, hold onto the base of the condom as you pull out to prevent any spills, then wrap it up and toss it in the trash. Easy peasy!

Types of Condoms:

Did you know there are loads of different types of condoms out there? From latex to non-latex, flavored to ribbed, there's something for everyone. If you or your partner has a latex allergy, no worries—

there are latex-free options available. And if you want to spice things up, why not try a flavored or textured condom for some extra fun?

Always Be Prepared:

One last thing—make sure you've always got condoms on hand whenever you're getting busy. Keep a stash in your bedside drawer, backpack, or purse so you're ready to roll whenever the mood strikes. And never be afraid to speak up and suggest using condoms—your health and safety are worth it!

Remember, using condoms isn't just about protecting yourself—it's about respecting yourself and your partner(s) and taking responsibility for your sexual health. So grab a condom, get consent, and get ready for some safe and satisfying fun!

Birth Control: Taking Charge of Your Reproductive Health

If you're getting down and dirty between the sheets and you're not quite ready for a baby, birth control is your new best friend. Let's dive into the world of birth control and explore your options for staying baby-free while still having fun.

Why Birth Control Matters:

First things first—if you're engaging in vaginal intercourse and you're not ready to become a parent, using birth control is absolutely essential. Birth control methods help prevent pregnancy by stopping sperm from fertilizing an egg or by preventing ovulation altogether. This means you can get jiggy with it without worrying about an unexpected bun in the oven.

Types of Birth Control:

The cool thing about birth control is that there are tons of options to choose from, so you can find one that fits your lifestyle and preferences. Hormonal methods, like the pill, patch, or contraceptive injection, work by releasing hormones into your body that prevent ovulation and thicken cervical mucus to block sperm. Non-hormonal methods, like the copper IUD, create an environment in your uterus that's hostile to sperm, preventing fertilization.

Finding the Right Fit:

When it comes to birth control, there's no one-size-fits-all solution. What works for your bestie might not work for you, and that's totally okay. Take some time to explore your options and talk to your healthcare provider about what might be the best choice for you. They can help you weigh the pros and cons of each method and find one that fits your needs and lifestyle.

Consistency is Key:

No matter what type of birth control you choose, the most important thing is to use it consistently and correctly. Missing a pill or forgetting to replace your patch can decrease its effectiveness, so it's crucial to stay on top of your birth control regimen. Set reminders on your phone, keep track of your pill pack, or explore long-acting options like the IUD or implant for hassle-free protection.

Double Up for Extra Protection:

Here's a pro tip—using condoms in addition to your chosen method of birth control can provide extra protection against both pregnancy and sexually transmitted infections (STIs). Plus, it's always better to be safe than sorry, right?

Final Thoughts:

Choosing a birth control method is an important decision, but it doesn't have to be overwhelming. Take your time, do your research, and don't be afraid to ask questions. With the right birth control method and some good old-fashioned communication with your partner, you can enjoy worry-free sex and take charge of your reproductive health like a boss.

Communication: Building Trust and Connection

When it comes to navigating the waters of safe sex, communication is your secret weapon. Open and honest conversations with your partner(s) can make all the difference in practicing safe and enjoyable sex. Let's dive into why communication is so important and how to make sure you're on the same page.

Why Communication Matters:

Communication forms the foundation of any healthy relationship, especially when it comes to sex. Talking openly about your sexual history, STI testing, and contraceptive preferences helps ensure that everyone involved is on the same page and can make informed decisions about their sexual health. Plus, discussing boundaries, consent, and mutual respect sets the stage for a positive and enjoyable sexual experience for everyone involved.

Starting the Conversation:

Bringing up topics like sexual health and boundaries can feel a bit awkward at first, but trust us—it's worth it. Find a quiet, comfortable time to chat with your partner(s) when you're both relaxed and open to discussion. You can start by sharing your own thoughts and feelings, then ask your partner(s) to do the same. Remember, communication is a two-way street, so be sure to listen as much as you talk.

Discussing Sexual History and STI Testing:

Sharing your sexual history and STI testing status with your partner(s) is an important step in protecting everyone's health. Be honest about your past experiences and any potential risks, and encourage your partner(s) to do the same. If either of you hasn't been tested recently, consider getting tested together—it's a great way to show you care about each other's well-being.

Talking About Contraceptive Preferences:

Discussing contraceptive preferences is another crucial aspect of sexual communication. Share your thoughts on birth control methods, condoms, and other forms of protection, and be open to your partner(s)'s preferences as well. Remember, it's okay to have different preferences, but it's important to find a solution that works for everyone involved.

Establishing Boundaries and Consent:

Setting boundaries and obtaining consent are non-negotiables when it comes to healthy and respectful sexual encounters. Talk with your partner(s) about what you're comfortable with and what you're not, and be sure to respect their boundaries as well. Remember, consent should be enthusiastic, ongoing, and freely given by all parties involved.

Final Thoughts:

Communication may not always be easy, but it's an essential part of practicing safe and enjoyable sex. By fostering open and honest conversations with your partner(s), you can build trust, deepen your connection, and ensure that everyone involved feels respected and valued. So don't be afraid to speak up and share your thoughts—you'll be glad you did.

STI Testing: Taking Control of Your Sexual Health

Getting tested for sexually transmitted infections (STIs) might not be the most glamorous part of sex, but it's a crucial step in protecting yourself and your partners. Let's break down why STI testing is so important and how you can make it a regular part of your sexual health routine.

Why STI Testing Matters:

STI testing is like hitting the refresh button on your sexual health—it's all about staying informed and taking proactive steps to protect yourself and your partners. Many STIs don't show any symptoms, which means you could have one without even knowing it. By getting tested regularly, you can catch any infections early and get the treatment you need to stay healthy.

Who Should Get Tested:

Everyone who's sexually active should consider getting tested for STIs, especially if you have multiple partners or engage in high-risk behaviors like unprotected sex or sharing needles. It's also a good idea to get tested before starting a new sexual relationship, even if you don't have any symptoms.

What to Expect During Testing:

STI testing might sound intimidating, but it's actually a pretty straightforward process. Depending on the type of STI you're getting tested for, you might need to provide a urine sample, a blood sample, or a swab from your genitals or mouth. Most STI tests are quick and painless, and you'll usually get your results within a few days.

Where to Get Tested:

You have several options for getting tested for STIs, including your healthcare provider, local clinics, or sexual health centers. Many colleges and universities also offer free or low-cost STI testing for students. If you're not sure where to go, do a quick Google search or ask your healthcare provider for recommendations.

The Importance of Regular Testing:

Getting tested for STIs should be a regular part of your sexual health routine, just like going to the dentist or getting your annual physical. Even if you feel fine and don't have any symptoms, it's still important to get tested regularly to stay on top of your sexual health and ensure peace of mind for you and your partners.

Final Thoughts:

STI testing might not be the most glamorous part of sex, but it's a crucial step in protecting yourself and your partners. By getting tested regularly and staying informed about your sexual health, you can enjoy a fulfilling and worry-free sex life while keeping yourself healthy and happy. So don't wait—schedule your STI test today and take control of your sexual health like a boss.

Consent: The Key to Respectful and Healthy Relationships

Consent is like the golden rule of sex—it's all about mutual respect, communication, and ensuring that everyone involved is on the same page. Let's dive into what consent really means and why it's so important for healthy and enjoyable sexual interactions.

What is Consent?

Consent is a clear and enthusiastic agreement to engage in sexual activity. It's not just about saying "yes" or "no"—it's about actively participating and freely choosing to engage in sexual activities without feeling pressured or coerced. Consent must be given willingly, without any manipulation or intimidation, and can be withdrawn at any time.

The Principles of Consent:

There are a few key principles that define what consent looks like in practice:

1. **Enthusiastic**: Consent should be enthusiastic and eager, showing genuine excitement and desire to participate in sexual activities.

2. **Ongoing**: Consent is not a one-time deal—it's an ongoing process that needs to be communicated and reaffirmed throughout the sexual encounter.

3. **Freely Given**: Consent must be given without any form of coercion, manipulation, or pressure. It should be a voluntary choice made without fear of consequences.

4. **Informed**: Consent requires clear communication and understanding of what's being agreed to. This means being

aware of the sexual activities involved and any potential risks or boundaries.

How to Practice Consent:

Practicing consent is all about open communication, active listening, and respecting each other's boundaries. Here are some tips for navigating consent in your sexual encounters:

- o **Ask for Consent**: Always ask for and receive verbal consent before engaging in sexual activities. This can be as simple as saying, "Are you okay with this?" or "Do you want to keep going?"

- o **Listen and Respect Boundaries**: Pay attention to your partner's verbal and non-verbal cues, and respect their boundaries and limits. If they say "no" or seem hesitant, stop immediately and check in with them.

- o **Communicate Openly**: Be open and honest with your partner(s) about your own boundaries, desires, and comfort levels. Encourage them to do the same, and create a safe space where everyone feels comfortable expressing themselves.

- o **Check In Regularly**: Consent isn't a one-time thing—it's an ongoing process. Check in with your partner(s) throughout your sexual encounter to make sure everyone is still comfortable and consenting to what's happening.

Final Thoughts:

Consent is the foundation of healthy and respectful sexual interactions. By practicing clear communication, active listening, and mutual respect, you can ensure that everyone involved feels safe, valued, and empowered in their sexual experiences. Remember, sex should be a positive and enjoyable experience for everyone, and consent is the key to making that happen. So always remember to ask for and respect consent—it's the right thing to do.

Safer Sex Practices: Taking Extra Steps for Your Well-being

While condoms and birth control are essential tools for protecting yourself during sex, there are additional steps you can take to enhance your safety and minimize risks. Let's explore some safer sex practices that can help you stay healthy and enjoy worry-free sexual encounters.

Avoid Sharing Needles or Injection Equipment:

Sharing needles or injection equipment can increase the risk of transmitting blood-borne infections like HIV and hepatitis. If you or your partner(s) use injectable drugs, it's crucial to use clean needles and equipment every time and never share them with others. Accessing needle exchange programs or seeking support for substance use can help reduce the risk of infection.

Use Dental Dams or Condoms for Oral Sex:

Oral sex can also transmit STIs like herpes, gonorrhea, and chlamydia, so it's important to use protection during oral encounters. Dental dams, which are thin latex or plastic barriers, can be used to cover the vagina or anus during oral-vaginal or oral-anal sex, while condoms can be used to cover the penis during oral-penile sex. Using protection during oral sex can help reduce the risk of STI transmission and keep you and your partner(s) safe.

Reduce Alcohol or Drug Use During Sexual Encounters:

Alcohol and drugs can impair judgment and lower inhibitions, leading to risky sexual behaviors and increased vulnerability to STIs and unwanted pregnancies. To minimize risks, consider limiting alcohol or drug use during sexual encounters and making decisions about consent and protection when you're sober and clear-headed. If you choose to drink or use drugs, do so responsibly and be mindful of your limits.

Communicate and Negotiate Safer Sex Practices:

Open communication with your partner(s) about safer sex practices is key to ensuring that everyone's needs and boundaries are respected. Discussing your preferences, concerns, and boundaries before engaging in sexual activities can help establish mutual understanding and trust. Be proactive in negotiating safer sex practices that work for both you and your partner(s), and be willing to adapt and adjust as needed.

Get Tested Regularly:

Regular STI testing is an essential part of safer sex practices, especially if you have multiple partners or engage in high-risk behaviors. Getting tested regularly allows you to stay informed about your sexual health status and take prompt action if you test positive for an STI. Many STI testing centers offer confidential and low-cost or free testing services, so don't hesitate to schedule a test and prioritize your well-being.

Final Thoughts:

Incorporating safer sex practices into your sexual activities can help reduce the risk of STI transmission, unwanted pregnancies, and other sexual health concerns. By being proactive, communicative, and mindful of your choices, you can enjoy fulfilling and worry-free sexual encounters while prioritizing your health and well-being. Remember, safer sex is smart sex, so take the necessary steps to protect yourself and your partner(s) every time.

Seeking Help and Resources: Your Guide to Sexual Health Support

Navigating sexual health concerns can sometimes feel overwhelming, but you're never alone in this journey. There are plenty of resources and support services available to help you address any questions or issues you may have. Let's explore some of the options for seeking help and finding the support you need.

1. Healthcare Providers:

Your healthcare provider is your go-to source for all things related to sexual health. Whether you have questions about birth control, STI testing, or sexual dysfunction, your doctor or gynecologist can offer expert advice, guidance, and medical treatment. Don't hesitate to schedule an appointment to discuss any concerns or issues you may have—it's their job to help you stay healthy and informed.

2. Sexual Health Clinics:

Sexual health clinics specialize in providing confidential and non-judgmental services related to sexual health. From STI testing and treatment to contraceptive counseling and reproductive health services, sexual health clinics offer a wide range of resources to meet your needs. Many clinics offer low-cost or free services, making them accessible to everyone regardless of income or insurance status.

3. Hotlines and Helplines:

If you have urgent questions or concerns about sexual health outside of regular business hours, hotlines and helplines are available to provide support and assistance. Organizations like Planned Parenthood and the Centers for Disease Control and

Prevention (CDC) offer toll-free hotlines staffed by trained professionals who can answer your questions, provide information, and offer support.

4. Online Resources:

The internet is a treasure trove of information on sexual health, with countless websites, forums, and resources available at your fingertips. Websites like Planned Parenthood, Scarleteen, and the American Sexual Health Association offer comprehensive information on topics ranging from contraception and STIs to sexual pleasure and consent. Just be sure to verify the credibility of the sources you're using and consult reputable websites for accurate and up-to-date information.

5. Support Groups:

Connecting with others who share similar experiences or concerns can be incredibly empowering and validating. Consider joining a support group or online community focused on sexual health topics like reproductive rights, LGBTQ+ issues, or living with STIs. These groups provide a safe space to share stories, ask questions, and receive support from others who understand what you're going through.

Final Thoughts:

When it comes to sexual health, seeking help and resources is a sign of strength, not weakness. Whether you have questions about contraception, STIs, or sexual pleasure, there are professionals and support services available to assist you every step of the way. Don't hesitate to reach out for help when you need it—you deserve to have access to accurate information, compassionate support, and quality care for your sexual health needs.

Conclusion: Prioritizing Your Sexual Health

Congratulations! You've reached the end of our journey through the world of safe sex and sexual health. We've covered a lot of ground—from using condoms and birth control to communicating effectively and seeking help when needed. Now, let's take a moment to reflect on what we've learned and how you can apply it to your own life.

Remember, your sexual health is a fundamental aspect of your overall well-being, and it's essential to prioritize it just like you would any other aspect of your health. By practicing safer sex habits, communicating openly with your partner(s), and seeking support when needed, you can take control of your sexual health and enjoy fulfilling and satisfying sexual experiences.

But sexual health isn't just about preventing STIs and unwanted pregnancies—it's also about embracing your sexuality, exploring your desires, and experiencing pleasure in a safe and consensual way. So don't be afraid to explore your own body, learn what feels good to you, and advocate for your own needs and desires.

Above all, remember that you are worthy of love, respect, and pleasure, and you have the right to make informed decisions about your own body and sexuality. Whether you're exploring new relationships, navigating sexual feelings, or seeking support for sexual health concerns, know that there are resources and support services available to assist you every step of the way.

So go forth with confidence, curiosity, and compassion, and remember that your sexual health journey is unique to you. Embrace it, learn from it, and always prioritize your well-being above all else.

Thank you for joining us on this journey through safe sex and sexual health. Here's to a lifetime of fulfilling, satisfying, and healthy sexual experiences. Cheers to you and your sexual health!

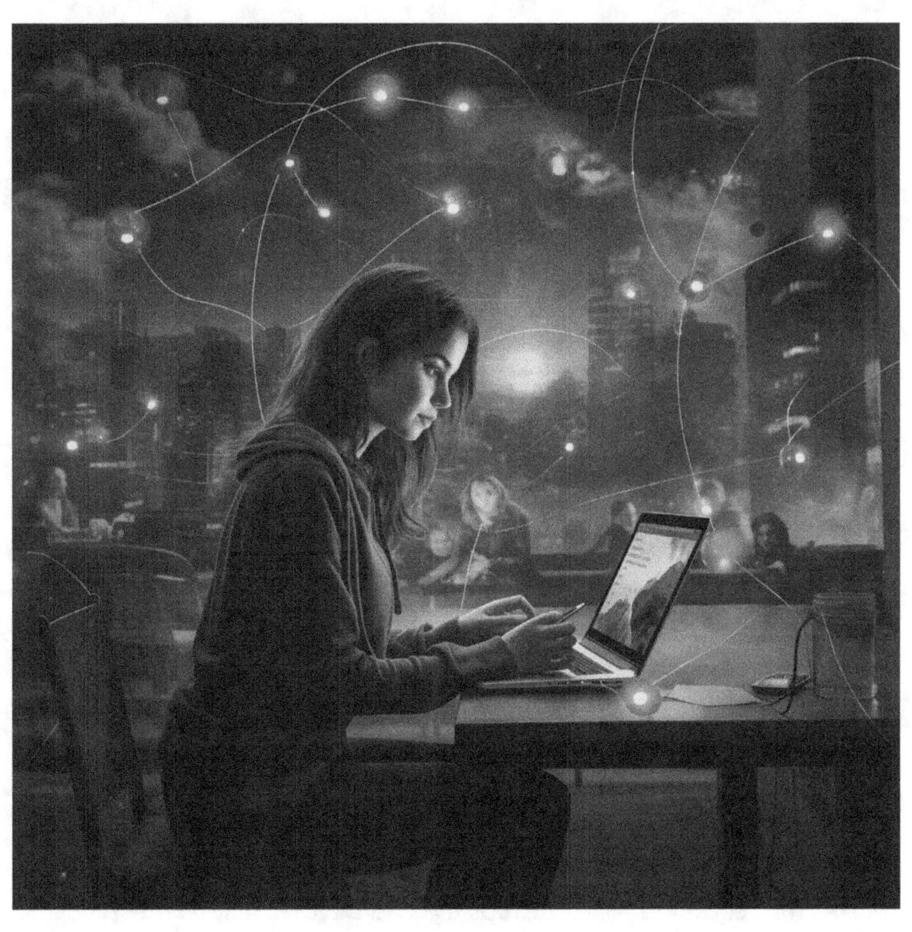

Chapter 8

Online Relationships and Safety

In our increasingly digital world, online relationships have become a common and integral part of how we connect with others. Whether it's through social media platforms, dating apps, or online forums, the internet offers a vast array of opportunities to form connections and build relationships.

In today's digital age, the prevalence of online relationships cannot be understated. With the rise of smartphones, high-speed internet, and social networking sites, people have more ways than ever to connect with others from all around the world. This accessibility has made online relationships a significant aspect of modern social interaction.

Online connections come in various forms, each offering its unique dynamics and opportunities for connection. From forging new friendships in online communities to exploring romantic connections on dating apps, the possibilities for forming relationships online are endless. Social media platforms like Facebook, Instagram, and Twitter provide avenues for maintaining connections with friends and family, sharing updates about our lives, and engaging in conversations on a global scale.

Furthermore, online relationships extend beyond just friendships and romantic connections. They also encompass professional networking, collaborative projects, and support networks for various interests and communities. Online forums, discussion groups, and virtual communities offer spaces for like-minded individuals to come together, share experiences, and support one another.

In essence, online relationships have become a fundamental aspect of how we interact and connect with others in the digital age. While they may differ from traditional face-to-face interactions in some ways, online relationships offer unique opportunities for communication, collaboration, and community-building. As we navigate the complexities of online connections, it's essential to approach them with an open mind, respect, and an understanding of the potential benefits and challenges they entail.

Embracing the Positivity: Understanding the Benefits of Online Connections

In today's digital age, online relationships have become an integral part of how we connect and interact with others. Beyond the convenience of instant communication, online connections offer a multitude of benefits that enrich our lives and broaden our horizons.

Accessibility Without Boundaries:

One of the most significant advantages of online connections is their unparalleled accessibility. Regardless of geographical barriers or physical limitations, individuals can forge connections with people from all corners of the globe. This accessibility fosters inclusivity and diversity, allowing individuals to engage with a wide range of perspectives and cultures that may not be readily available in their immediate surroundings.

Community Building and Shared Interests:

Online platforms serve as virtual hubs for community building, where individuals with shared interests can come together to connect, collaborate, and celebrate their passions. Whether it's a subreddit dedicated to a specific hobby, a Facebook group for local enthusiasts, or an online forum for fans of a particular TV show, these digital communities foster a sense of belonging and camaraderie among like-minded individuals. Through these platforms, individuals can find support, inspiration, and a sense of belonging that transcends physical boundaries.

Support and Solidarity:

For marginalized or isolated individuals, online connections can be a lifeline, offering much-needed support, companionship, and validation. Online support groups provide safe spaces for individuals facing similar challenges to share their experiences, seek advice, and offer mutual support. Whether it's a forum for mental health support, a social media group for LGBTQ+ youth, or an online community for survivors of trauma, these digital spaces offer solace and solidarity to those who may feel marginalized or alone in their offline lives.

Unconditional Acceptance and Understanding:

In the digital realm, individuals have the freedom to express themselves authentically without fear of judgment or discrimination. Online connections can provide a sense of acceptance and understanding that may be lacking in offline interactions. Whether it's finding solidarity with others who share similar experiences or receiving words of encouragement from virtual friends, online relationships offer a refuge where individuals can be their true selves without reservation.

In essence, online connections offer a wealth of benefits that enhance our lives in profound and meaningful ways. From fostering a sense of community and belonging to providing support and solidarity in times of need, online relationships enrich our lives and expand our perspectives. By embracing the positive aspects of online connections and fostering a culture of respect, empathy, and inclusivity, we can harness the transformative power of the digital realm to build stronger, more connected communities.

Navigating the Hazards: Understanding Challenges and Risks in Online Relationships

As we delve deeper into the realm of online relationships, it's crucial to acknowledge the challenges and risks that come hand in hand with this digital landscape. While online connections offer a plethora of benefits, they also present a range of potential pitfalls that can impact our mental health and well-being.

Cyberbullying and Online Harassment:

One of the most prevalent risks associated with online relationships is the threat of cyberbullying and online harassment. In the anonymity of the digital world, individuals may feel emboldened to engage in hurtful behavior, such as spreading rumors, making derogatory comments, or sending threatening messages. Cyberbullying can have devastating effects on its victims, leading to feelings of fear, anxiety, and low self-esteem. It's essential to be vigilant and proactive in addressing instances of cyberbullying and creating safe online spaces where individuals can feel protected and supported.

Privacy Concerns and Data Security:

Another significant risk in online relationships is the potential for privacy breaches and data security threats. With the widespread use of social media platforms and online communication tools, individuals may inadvertently share sensitive personal information that can be exploited by malicious actors. From identity theft to online scams and phishing attacks, the internet poses numerous risks to our privacy and security. It's crucial to exercise caution when sharing personal information online and to be aware of the privacy settings and security measures offered by online platforms.

Impact on Mental Health and Well-being:

Furthermore, online interactions can have a profound impact on our mental health and well-being. The constant exposure to curated images and idealized lifestyles on social media platforms can contribute to feelings of inadequacy, comparison, and self-doubt. Moreover, the lack of face-to-face interaction in online relationships can exacerbate feelings of loneliness, isolation, and disconnection from real-life social networks. It's essential to be mindful of the emotional toll that online interactions can take and to prioritize self-care and digital well-being practices to maintain a healthy balance between our online and offline lives.

In essence, while online relationships offer a wealth of opportunities for connection and community, they also come with inherent risks and challenges that must be navigated with care and caution. By being aware of these potential pitfalls and taking proactive steps to mitigate them, we can cultivate safer and more fulfilling online experiences that contribute positively to our mental health and overall well-being.

Building Strong Foundations: Nurturing Healthy Online Relationships

In the vast landscape of the digital world, cultivating healthy online relationships requires intentionality, empathy, and a commitment to fostering positive interactions. Let's explore strategies for nurturing strong and respectful connections in the digital realm, while maintaining a healthy balance between our online and offline lives.

Effective Communication:

Effective communication lies at the heart of healthy relationships, both online and offline. In the digital realm, where tone and nuance can easily be misinterpreted, clear and transparent communication is paramount. This involves expressing ourselves honestly and respectfully, actively listening to others' perspectives, and being mindful of our words and actions. By fostering open and honest dialogue, we can build trust, understanding, and mutual respect in our online interactions.

Setting Boundaries:

Setting boundaries is essential for maintaining healthy online relationships and protecting our well-being. Boundaries help establish clear expectations and guidelines for how we engage with others online, including what content we share, how we respond to messages, and when we disconnect. By establishing and communicating our boundaries clearly and assertively, we can create a safe and respectful environment for ourselves and others in the digital space.

Practicing Empathy:

Empathy is a cornerstone of healthy relationships, allowing us to understand and validate others' experiences, emotions, and perspectives. In the digital realm, where interactions often lack face-to-face cues, empathy plays a crucial role in bridging the gap and fostering meaningful connections. By putting ourselves in others' shoes, actively listening to their concerns, and responding with compassion and understanding, we can cultivate empathy in our online interactions and build deeper, more authentic relationships.

Balancing Online and Offline Interactions:

While online relationships offer opportunities for connection and community, it's essential to maintain a healthy balance between our digital and offline lives. Spending excessive time online can lead to feelings of isolation, burnout, and disconnection from real-life social networks. Therefore, it's crucial to prioritize face-to-face interactions, engage in offline activities that bring us joy and fulfillment, and take breaks from social media when needed. By striking a balance between our online and offline worlds, we can ensure that our digital interactions enhance rather than detract from our overall well-being.

Combatting Cyberbullying: Strategies for Prevention and Response

In the digital age, cyberbullying has emerged as a pervasive and harmful phenomenon, threatening the well-being and safety of individuals in online spaces. Let's delve into the definition of cyberbullying, its various forms, and strategies for both prevention and response to ensure the safety and security of online communities.

Understanding Cyberbullying:

Cyberbullying encompasses a range of harmful behaviors perpetrated online, including harassment, trolling, cyberstalking, and impersonation. These actions can take many forms, such as sending threatening or abusive messages, spreading rumors or false information, posting derogatory comments or images, and creating fake accounts to impersonate or harass others. Cyberbullying can have devastating effects on its victims, leading to feelings of fear, anxiety, depression, and low self-esteem. It's essential to recognize the signs of cyberbullying and take proactive steps to address and prevent it.

Recognizing and Responding to Cyberbullying:

Recognizing and responding to cyberbullying requires vigilance, empathy, and a commitment to creating safe and inclusive online spaces. If you or someone you know is experiencing cyberbullying, it's essential to take action promptly and assertively. This may involve blocking or unfriending the perpetrator, documenting evidence of the abusive behavior, and reporting it to the appropriate authorities or online platforms. Additionally, seeking support from trusted adults, friends, or mental health professionals can provide much-needed guidance and assistance in navigating the situation.

Prevention Through Education and Empowerment:

Preventing cyberbullying requires a multi-faceted approach that addresses root causes and promotes positive digital citizenship. Educating individuals about the impact of cyberbullying, fostering empathy and respect in online interactions, and promoting responsible use of technology are crucial steps in preventing cyberbullying from occurring in the first place. Empowering individuals to speak out against cyberbullying, support those who are affected, and cultivate safe and inclusive online communities is essential for creating a digital environment where everyone can thrive.

Reporting and Seeking Support:

If you encounter cyberbullying or witness abusive behavior online, it's essential to take action by reporting it to the appropriate authorities or online platforms. Most social media platforms and online communities have mechanisms in place for reporting abusive behavior, such as reporting tools, helplines, or support resources. By reporting cyberbullying and seeking support from trusted adults or online platforms, we can work together to combat cyberbullying and create a safer and more respectful online environment for all.

Securing Your Digital Fortress: Essential Online Safety Practices

In the vast expanse of the digital world, safeguarding your personal information and online identity is paramount to ensuring a secure and positive online experience. Let's explore practical tips and strategies for enhancing your online safety and protecting yourself from potential threats and risks.

Protecting Personal Information:

One of the first lines of defense in online safety is safeguarding your personal information from prying eyes and malicious actors. This includes using strong, unique passwords for your online accounts, enabling two-factor authentication whenever possible, and refraining from sharing sensitive details such as your full name, address, phone number, or financial information with strangers or untrusted sources. By exercising caution and discretion when sharing personal information online, you can minimize the risk of identity theft, fraud, and other forms of cybercrime.

Navigating Online Interactions with Caution:

When interacting with unfamiliar individuals online, it's essential to approach with caution and skepticism. While the digital realm offers opportunities for connection and community, it also presents risks of encountering fraudulent or deceptive individuals. Be wary of requests for personal information or financial assistance from strangers, and take steps to verify the authenticity of online contacts before engaging further. Trust your instincts and err on the side of caution when in doubt, as your safety and security should always take precedence in online interactions.

Enhancing Privacy and Security Settings:

Maximizing your privacy and security settings on online platforms and social media accounts is another crucial aspect of online safety. Take the time to review and adjust your privacy settings to control who can view your profile, posts, and personal information. Regularly update your devices and software to patch security vulnerabilities and protect against malware, viruses, and other cyber threats. By staying proactive and vigilant in managing your online privacy and security settings, you can minimize the risk of unauthorized access to your personal information and digital assets.

Educating Yourself and Others:

Finally, staying informed and educated about online safety practices is key to navigating the digital landscape with confidence and resilience. Take advantage of resources and educational materials available online, such as cybersecurity guides, tutorials, and webinars, to deepen your understanding of online threats and best practices for staying safe online. Share your knowledge and insights with friends, family members, and peers to empower them to take proactive steps towards enhancing their own online safety and security.

Guarding Against Danger: Identifying Red Flags of Online Predators

In the vast expanse of the digital world, where connections are forged with the click of a button, it's essential to remain vigilant and aware of potential threats lurking in the shadows. Online predators, individuals who seek to exploit and harm others, often use manipulative tactics to groom and prey on unsuspecting victims. Let's explore common signs and red flags of online predatory behavior to help you recognize and avoid potential dangers.

Understanding Predatory Tactics:

Online predators employ a range of manipulative tactics to gain the trust and compliance of their victims. These tactics may include flattery, persuasion, manipulation, and coercion to lure victims into harmful situations. By exploiting vulnerabilities and insecurities, online predators aim to establish control over their victims and exploit them for their own gratification or gain.

Recognizing Warning Signs:

There are several warning signs and red flags that may indicate predatory behavior in online interactions. These include:

1. Requests for inappropriate or explicit photos or videos.

2. Attempts to isolate the victim from friends, family, or support networks.

3. Manipulative tactics, such as guilt-tripping, gaslighting, or love-bombing.

4. Pressure to engage in sexual activities or meet in person against your will.

5. Refusal to respect boundaries or take no for an answer.

6. Attempts to gain access to personal information or private accounts.

Protecting Yourself and Others:

To protect yourself and others from online predators, it's crucial to remain vigilant and trust your instincts. If you encounter any suspicious or concerning behavior online, trust your gut and take proactive steps to protect yourself. This may involve blocking or unfriending the individual, reporting their behavior to the appropriate authorities or online platforms, and seeking support from trusted friends, family members, or mental health professionals.

Promoting Awareness and Education:

Additionally, promoting awareness and education about online predatory behavior is essential for empowering individuals to recognize and respond to potential dangers. Educate yourself and others about the tactics used by online predators, and share information about warning signs and red flags to watch out for in online interactions. By fostering a culture of vigilance, awareness, and support, we can work together to create safer and more inclusive online communities for everyone.

In conclusion, recognizing red flags of online predatory behavior is crucial for safeguarding yourself and others from potential harm in the digital world. By understanding predatory tactics, recognizing warning signs, and taking proactive steps to protect yourself and promote awareness, you can navigate online interactions with confidence and resilience, ensuring a safer and more secure digital experience for all.

Empowering Your Digital Savvy: Harnessing Critical Thinking and Digital Literacy

In today's digital landscape, where information flows freely and connections are forged in virtual realms, the ability to think critically and navigate the digital terrain with discernment is more crucial than ever. Let's delve into the importance of developing critical thinking skills and digital literacy to navigate online relationships safely, along with practical tips for evaluating online content and avoiding common pitfalls.

The Power of Critical Thinking:

Critical thinking is the cornerstone of digital literacy, empowering individuals to question, analyze, and evaluate information critically. In the age of information overload, being able to discern fact from fiction, identify bias, and recognize potential misinformation is essential for making informed decisions and navigating the digital landscape safely. By honing your critical thinking skills, you can become a more discerning and empowered consumer of online content, better equipped to navigate the complexities of the digital world with confidence and clarity.

Navigating the Digital Terrain:

In the vast sea of online content, discerning fact from fiction can be a daunting task. However, with the right tools and strategies, you can navigate the digital terrain with ease and confidence. Start by critically evaluating the source and credibility of online content, considering factors such as authorship, expertise, and potential bias. Be skeptical of sensationalized headlines, clickbait, and misinformation, and take the time to verify information through reputable sources before sharing or acting upon it.

Avoiding Scams and Fraudulent Activities:

In addition to discerning misinformation, developing digital literacy skills is crucial for avoiding scams, fraudulent activities, and online threats. Be wary of unsolicited messages, emails, or requests for personal information, and never provide sensitive details such as passwords, financial information, or social security numbers to untrusted sources. Familiarize yourself with common online scams and phishing tactics, and take proactive steps to protect yourself and your personal information from potential threats.

Promoting Digital Citizenship:

Ultimately, developing critical thinking skills and digital literacy is not just about protecting yourself—it's also about promoting responsible digital citizenship and contributing positively to online communities. Be mindful of your online behavior and interactions, respect the privacy and rights of others, and engage in online discussions and debates with civility and respect. By fostering a culture of critical thinking, digital literacy, and responsible digital citizenship, we can create safer, more inclusive, and more informed online communities for everyone.

Throughout this chapter, we've embarked on a journey through the digital frontier, exploring the intricacies of online relationships, the challenges of cyber interactions, and the importance of safety and well-being in the digital realm. Let's take a moment to recap the key points covered and reflect on the insights gained.

Embracing the Benefits and Acknowledging the Risks:

In our exploration of online relationships, we've encountered a myriad of benefits, from the accessibility and community-building opportunities offered by digital connections to the support and companionship they provide, particularly for marginalized or isolated individuals. However, we've also recognized the risks and challenges inherent in the digital landscape, from cyberbullying and online harassment to the threat of online predators and scams.

Strategies for Building Healthy Connections:

Amidst the complexities of online interactions, we've uncovered strategies for building healthy and respectful connections in the digital realm. By prioritizing effective communication, setting boundaries, practicing empathy, and maintaining a healthy balance between online and offline interactions, we can cultivate fulfilling relationships that enrich our lives and contribute positively to our digital well-being.

Tips for Staying Safe Online:

In our quest for digital empowerment, we've equipped ourselves with practical tips and strategies for staying safe online. From protecting personal information and enhancing privacy settings to recognizing red flags of online predatory behavior and promoting digital literacy and critical thinking, we've fortified our defenses and empowered ourselves to navigate the digital landscape with confidence and resilience.

Final Thoughts:

As we conclude our exploration of online relationships and safety, let us reaffirm the importance of prioritizing safety and well-being in all our digital interactions. The digital world offers boundless opportunities for connection, creativity, and collaboration, but it also presents risks and challenges that must be navigated with care and caution. By applying the knowledge and insights gained from this chapter, we can embark on our digital journey with confidence, resilience, and a commitment to fostering safe, respectful, and inclusive online communities for all.

In essence, as we navigate the ever-evolving digital landscape, let us remember to prioritize safety, well-being, and respect in all our online interactions. By fostering empathy, practicing critical thinking, and promoting digital citizenship, we can create a digital world that is safer, more inclusive, and more empowering for everyone. Together, let us embark on this journey with courage, compassion, and a steadfast commitment to building a better digital future for all.

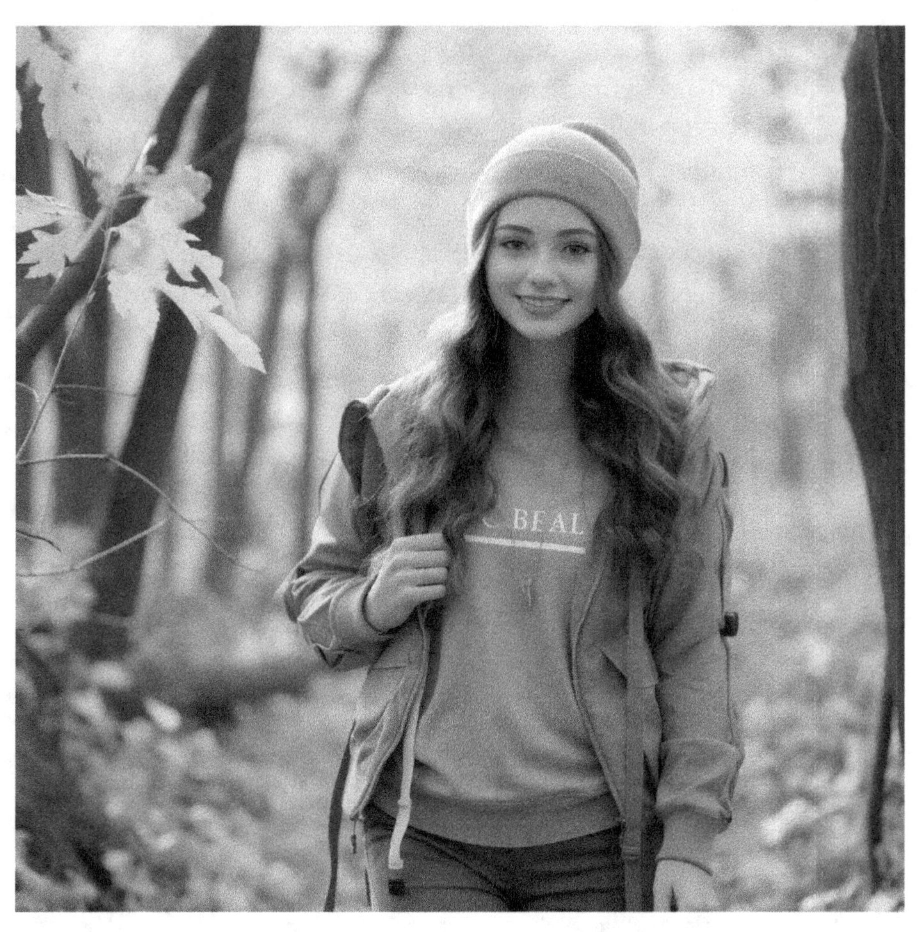

Chapter 9

Self-Care and Well-Being

In today's fast-paced and demanding world, the concept of self-care and well-being has become increasingly relevant. But what exactly do we mean by self-care and well-being, and why are they so crucial in our lives?

Self-care encompasses a broad spectrum of practices aimed at preserving and enhancing our mental, emotional, and physical health. It involves taking deliberate actions to nurture ourselves, recharge our batteries, and cultivate a sense of balance and harmony in our lives. Well-being, on the other hand, refers to our overall state of health and happiness, encompassing not just the absence of illness, but also the presence of positive emotions, fulfillment, and purpose.

The interconnectedness of mental, emotional, and physical health cannot be overstated. When one aspect of our well-being is compromised, it often affects other areas of our lives as well. In today's society, stress, burnout, and mental health challenges have become increasingly prevalent, fueled by factors such as work pressures, societal expectations, and the constant onslaught of information and stimuli.

In light of these challenges, self-care emerges as a vital tool for mitigating the negative effects of stress and promoting overall well-being. By prioritizing self-care, we empower ourselves to proactively manage our health and happiness, rather than simply reacting to external stressors. It is a proactive approach to self-preservation, a recognition of our own worth and value, and a commitment to nurturing ourselves amidst the demands of daily life.

As we embark on this journey through the realm of self-care and well-being, let us set the tone for the chapter by emphasizing the significance of prioritizing self-care. By investing in our own well-being, we not only enhance our quality of life but also empower ourselves to navigate life's challenges with resilience, vitality, and grace. So let us explore the transformative power of self-care and embark on a journey towards greater health, happiness, and fulfillment.

Self-care is not just about pampering oneself with bubble baths and spa days; it encompasses a holistic approach to nurturing one's well-being across various dimensions. It involves attending to our physical, emotional, social, and spiritual needs, recognizing that each aspect contributes to our overall health and happiness.

At its core, self-care is an act of self-compassion and self-respect. It's about recognizing our worth and prioritizing our needs, even amidst the demands of daily life. Contrary to popular belief, self-care is not selfish; it's essential for maintaining resilience, productivity, and overall happiness.

By investing in self-care, we equip ourselves with the tools to navigate life's challenges with grace and fortitude. Whether it's practicing mindfulness to cultivate inner peace, engaging in regular exercise to boost physical health, or setting boundaries to protect our emotional well-being, self-care empowers us to show up fully for ourselves and others.

Self-care practices can take many forms, depending on individual preferences and needs. It might involve taking time for hobbies and activities that bring joy, nourishing our bodies with nutritious foods, or seeking support from friends and loved ones when needed. Ultimately, self-care is about listening to our innermost needs and honoring them with compassion and kindness.

As we delve deeper into the concept of self-care, let us challenge the misconception that it is selfish or indulgent. Instead, let us recognize its role as a fundamental aspect of maintaining overall health and well-being. By embracing self-care, we not only enhance our own lives but also create a ripple effect of positivity and resilience in the world around us.

Prioritizing self-care isn't just a luxury reserved for spa days and relaxation; it's a crucial investment in our overall well-being. By taking deliberate steps to nurture ourselves, we reap a myriad of benefits that extend far beyond the surface. Let's explore some of the remarkable advantages of making self-care a priority in our lives.

Improved Mental and Emotional Health: Self-care practices such as mindfulness meditation, journaling, and therapy provide essential tools for managing stress, anxiety, and depression. By nurturing our mental and emotional well-being, we build resilience and develop healthier coping mechanisms to navigate life's challenges.

Reduced Stress Levels: Chronic stress takes a toll on our bodies and minds, leading to a host of health issues and diminished quality of life. Prioritizing self-care allows us to unwind, recharge, and restore balance, thereby reducing our overall stress levels and promoting a sense of calm and relaxation.

Enhanced Productivity: Contrary to popular belief, self-care is not a hindrance to productivity; it's a catalyst for it. When we take care of ourselves, we replenish our energy reserves and sharpen our focus, enabling us to work more efficiently and effectively. By incorporating self-care into our routine, we set ourselves up for success in both our personal and professional lives.

Better Relationships: Self-care isn't just about nurturing ourselves; it's also about fostering healthier relationships with others. When we prioritize our well-being, we show up as our best selves in our interactions with friends, family, and colleagues. We're more present, compassionate, and empathetic, leading to deeper connections and more fulfilling relationships.

Real-Life Stories and Testimonials: Countless individuals have experienced the transformative power of self-care in their own lives. From overcoming burnout and anxiety to rediscovering joy and fulfillment, their stories serve as a testament to the profound impact of prioritizing self-care. These real-life examples inspire and motivate us to prioritize our own well-being.

Research Findings and Studies: The benefits of self-care are not just anecdotal; they're backed by scientific research. Studies have shown that self-care practices such as exercise, adequate sleep, and social connection have a positive impact on mental health, physical health, and overall quality of life. These findings provide empirical evidence of the importance of self-care in promoting well-being.

In conclusion, prioritizing self-care is not selfish; it's essential. By investing in our own well-being, we not only improve our quality of life but also enhance our ability to show up fully for ourselves and others. Let's embrace self-care as a fundamental aspect of living a fulfilling and balanced life, and reap the multitude of benefits it brings.

Barriers to Self-Care

Despite the undeniable benefits of self-care, many individuals encounter barriers that hinder their ability to prioritize their well-being. Let's explore some common obstacles and strategies for overcoming them, empowering readers to make self-care a non-negotiable part of their lives.

Time Constraints: In today's busy world, time is often perceived as a scarce resource. Juggling work, family obligations, and social commitments leaves little room for self-care. However, it's essential to recognize that self-care doesn't have to be time-consuming. Even small, intentional acts of self-care can make a significant difference. Prioritize self-care by scheduling it into your daily routine, even if it's just a few minutes of mindfulness meditation or a short walk outside.

Guilt: Many individuals struggle with feelings of guilt when it comes to prioritizing their own needs. They may feel selfish or indulgent for taking time for themselves, especially when there are others depending on them. However, it's crucial to recognize that self-care is not selfish; it's a necessary investment in your well-being. Reframe self-care as a vital aspect of self-preservation, enabling you to show up more fully for others.

Societal Expectations: Society often glorifies busyness and productivity, equating self-care with laziness or weakness. However, challenging these societal norms is essential for prioritizing your well-being. Recognize that self-care is a fundamental human need, not a luxury reserved for the privileged few. Set boundaries and assertively communicate your needs to others, prioritizing your well-being without apology.

Internalized Beliefs: Internalized beliefs about worthiness and deservingness can sabotage our efforts to practice self-care. Negative self-talk and perfectionism may convince us that we're not deserving of self-care or that we don't have time for it. Challenge these limiting beliefs by cultivating self-compassion and self-acceptance. Remind yourself that you are worthy of love and care, and prioritize your well-being accordingly.

To overcome these barriers, it's essential to approach self-care with intentionality and self-compassion. Start by identifying your unique obstacles to self-care and brainstorming strategies for overcoming them. Lean on your support network for encouragement and accountability, and be gentle with yourself as you navigate the journey towards prioritizing your well-being. Remember, self-care isn't selfish—it's an act of self-love and self-preservation that benefits not only you but also those around you.

Cultivating a Self-Care Routine

Creating a self-care routine tailored to your unique needs and preferences is a powerful way to prioritize your well-being and nurture your mind, body, and spirit. Let's explore practical steps for developing a personalized self-care plan that supports your overall health and happiness.

Identify Your Self-Care Activities: Start by reflecting on activities that bring you joy, relaxation, and fulfillment. These can vary widely from person to person and may include hobbies, exercise, creative pursuits, mindfulness practices, or spending time in nature. Consider what activities recharge your energy and leave you feeling refreshed and invigorated.

Schedule Time for Self-Care: Once you've identified your self-care activities, integrate them into your daily or weekly schedule. Treat self-care appointments with the same level of importance as other commitments, and block out dedicated time for self-care in your calendar. Whether it's a morning meditation session, an afternoon walk, or an evening bath, prioritize self-care as non-negotiable time for yourself.

Create a Self-Care Plan: Develop a structured self-care plan that outlines your chosen activities, frequency, and duration. Consider creating a self-care checklist or journal to track your progress and hold yourself accountable. Be flexible and open to adjusting your self-care routine as needed to accommodate changes in your schedule or preferences.

Evaluate Your Progress: Regularly assess how your self-care routine is working for you. Pay attention to how you feel physically, emotionally, and mentally after engaging in self-care activities. Notice any patterns or trends in your well-being and adjust your self-care plan accordingly. Remember that self-care is an ongoing process of self-discovery and experimentation.

Emphasize Consistency and Self-Reflection: Consistency is key to maintaining a sustainable self-care practice. Aim to incorporate self-care into your daily or weekly routine, even on busy days when time is limited. Prioritize self-care as an essential aspect of your overall well-being, and make it a non-negotiable part of your lifestyle. Additionally, practice self-reflection to deepen your understanding of your needs and preferences. Take time to check in with yourself regularly and adjust your self-care routine as necessary.

By cultivating a personalized self-care routine, you empower yourself to prioritize your well-being and create a life that is balanced, fulfilling, and aligned with your values and goals. Remember that self-care is not selfish; it's a necessary investment in your health and happiness. So carve out time for yourself, honor your needs, and embrace the transformative power of self-care in your life.

Throughout this chapter, we've explored the vital role that self-care plays in maintaining overall well-being and navigating the challenges of daily life. From defining self-care to identifying common barriers and strategies for cultivating a personalized self-care routine, we've delved into the essential components of prioritizing our own health and happiness.

Self-care is not a luxury; it's a necessity—a fundamental aspect of nurturing our mental, emotional, and physical well-being. By taking deliberate steps to care for ourselves, we not only replenish our energy reserves but also build resilience and enhance our ability to cope with life's stressors.

We've discussed the importance of recognizing and overcoming barriers to self-care, such as time constraints, guilt, and societal expectations. By reframing self-care as a non-negotiable aspect of our daily routine and cultivating self-compassion and self-acceptance, we can overcome these obstacles and prioritize our well-being.

Creating a self-care routine that aligns with our individual preferences, needs, and goals empowers us to take ownership of our health and happiness. By incorporating self-care activities into our daily lives, scheduling dedicated time for self-care, and evaluating our progress regularly, we lay the foundation for a sustainable and fulfilling self-care practice.

As we conclude this chapter, I encourage you to prioritize your well-being by embracing self-care as an essential part of your life. Take proactive steps towards nurturing your mental, emotional, and physical health, and remember that self-care is not selfish—it's an act of self-love and self-preservation. By investing in yourself, you empower yourself to lead a life that is balanced, resilient, and deeply fulfilling. Embrace the journey towards holistic well-being through self-care practices, and may you find strength, empowerment, and joy along the way.

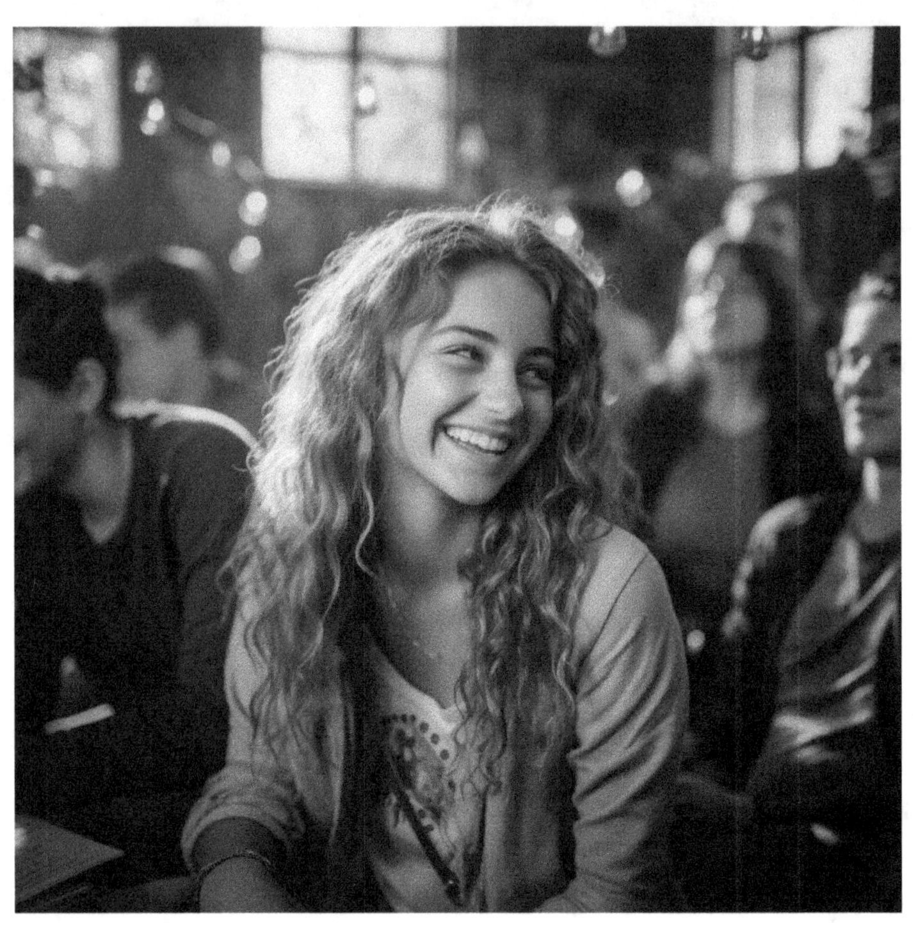

Chapter 10

Your Sexual Roadmap: Navigating Teen Years and Beyond

Welcome to the concluding chapter of our journey together! As we embark on this final stage of exploration, we'll delve into the significance of navigating one's sexual journey through adolescence and beyond.

Throughout this book, we've delved into various aspects of sexual health, relationships, and personal growth, aiming to equip you with knowledge, skills, and empowerment to navigate the complexities of sexuality with confidence and resilience.

In this final chapter, we'll reflect on the progress you've made, celebrate your achievements, and provide guidance for the road ahead. As you continue your journey, we'll explore the importance of setting goals, embracing diversity, advocating for rights, and overcoming challenges.

Navigating your sexual journey is not just about reaching a destination; it's about embracing the twists and turns, the highs and lows, and the moments of growth and self-discovery along the way. It's about recognizing that your journey is uniquely yours, and that each step you take is an opportunity for learning and growth.

So, let's embark on this final stage of exploration together, as we navigate the winding paths of adolescence and beyond, armed with knowledge, resilience, and a commitment to personal empowerment. Together, let's chart a course toward a future of sexual health, happiness, and fulfillment.

Reflecting on Personal Growth: Navigating Your Sexual Journey

As we near the end of our journey together, it's essential to take a moment to pause and reflect on how far you've come. Your journey of sexual exploration and self-discovery has been filled with moments of growth, challenges, and triumphs, each contributing to the person you are today.

Take a moment to think back to the beginning of this journey. Recall the questions, uncertainties, and curiosities that initially propelled you forward. Consider the knowledge you've gained, the insights you've discovered, and the new perspectives you've embraced along the way.

Reflect on the milestones you've reached—the conversations you've had, the boundaries you've set, and the decisions you've made about your sexual health and relationships. Celebrate the moments of courage, vulnerability, and authenticity that have shaped your journey and propelled you forward.

But reflection isn't just about looking back—it's also about looking forward. As you reflect on your personal growth, consider the lessons you've learned and how you can apply them to the future. Think about the goals you've set, the values you hold dear, and the vision you have for your sexual journey moving forward.

Reflecting on your personal growth is an opportunity to honor your journey, acknowledge your progress, and recognize the resilience and strength within you. It's a reminder that growth is a continuous process, and that each step you take is a testament to your courage and determination.

So, take a moment to pause and reflect on your journey thus far. Celebrate your growth, embrace your authenticity, and envision the bright future that lies ahead. Your journey of sexual exploration and self-discovery is a testament to your resilience, your strength, and your unwavering commitment to personal empowerment.

Celebrating Your Journey: Recognizing Milestones and Triumphs

In this final chapter, we pause to celebrate the incredible milestones and achievements you've attained in your journey toward sexual health and well-being. Your path has been marked by moments of courage, growth, and resilience, and each step forward deserves to be acknowledged and honored.

Take a moment to reflect on the progress you've made since beginning this journey. Perhaps you've educated yourself about sexual health topics, delving into resources and information to gain a deeper understanding of your body, relationships, and sexual well-being. Maybe you've engaged in open conversations with trusted individuals, breaking down taboos and fostering healthier communication about sex and relationships.

Consider the decisions you've made to prioritize your sexual health, whether it's practicing safer sex, seeking out contraception options, or advocating for your needs and boundaries in relationships. These choices reflect your commitment to self-care, self-respect, and empowerment.

Beyond tangible achievements, celebrate the moments of personal growth and self-discovery you've experienced. Embrace the times you've challenged societal norms, embraced diversity, and embraced your authentic self. These moments of authenticity and self-acceptance are just as vital to your journey as any external milestone.

As you celebrate your journey, also acknowledge the challenges you've faced—the doubts, fears, and uncertainties that once seemed insurmountable. Yet here you are, standing strong and resilient, having overcome those obstacles with grace and determination.

Looking ahead, let this celebration be a reminder of your strength and resilience as you continue to navigate your sexual journey. Each day presents new opportunities for growth, learning, and self-discovery. Embrace the journey, cherish your accomplishments, and know that you are worthy of every success that comes your way.

So, here's to you—to your courage, your resilience, and your unwavering commitment to prioritizing your sexual health and well-being. May you continue to celebrate your achievements, embrace your journey, and thrive in every aspect of your life. You've come so far, and the best is yet to come. Cheers to you and all that you've achieved!

Mapping Your Path Forward: Embracing the Journey of Growth

As we come to the end of this exploration together, it's essential to take a moment to gaze into the horizon of your future. Just as a map guides a traveler, setting goals for your sexual health and relationships can provide direction and purpose in your journey ahead.

But how do we embark on this journey of goal-setting with confidence and clarity? Let's navigate through this process together:

Reflect on Your Aspirations: Begin by contemplating your values and desires concerning your sexual health and relationships. What are the aspirations that reside within you? What future do you envision for yourself in these realms?

Identify Areas for Growth: Consider the facets of your sexual well-being and relationships where you aspire to grow. Perhaps it's fostering deeper communication with partners, cultivating greater self-confidence, or exploring new dimensions of your sexuality.

Crafting Your Vision: Formulate goals that are specific, meaningful, and attainable. Rather than setting broad objectives like "improving communication," aim for targeted outcomes such as "nurturing open dialogue through regular, honest conversations with my partner."

Break It Down: Break down larger aspirations into smaller, actionable steps. This approach not only renders your objectives more manageable but also celebrates the journey of progress with each accomplished milestone.

Flexibility and Adaptation: Be open to adaptation along your journey. Life's landscape is ever-changing, and your goals should evolve in harmony with your experiences and evolving priorities.

Embrace Support: Seek support from allies who champion your growth. Whether it's friends, family, or professionals, surrounding yourself with a supportive network can fuel your journey with encouragement and insight.

Celebrate Every Stride: Remember to acknowledge and celebrate each step forward. Every effort, no matter how modest, is a testament to your commitment and resilience.

By charting your course with intention and purpose, you empower yourself to navigate the intricate terrain of your sexual journey with confidence and clarity. Embrace the voyage, honor your progress, and revel in the infinite possibilities that lie ahead. Your journey is a testament to your courage, your resilience, and your unwavering dedication to crafting a future brimming with fulfillment and joy.

Celebrating Sexual Diversity: Embracing Inclusivity in Every Corner

In our journey toward understanding sexual health and relationships, one crucial aspect that demands our attention is the celebration of sexual diversity. Embracing inclusivity in all its forms is not just a moral imperative; it's a fundamental aspect of creating a world where everyone feels seen, valued, and respected.

At the heart of embracing sexual diversity lies the recognition that human sexuality is as diverse and multifaceted as the individuals who embody it. It encompasses a spectrum of identities, orientations, and expressions that defy rigid categorizations and binaries. From heterosexual to homosexual, bisexual, pansexual, asexual, and beyond, each identity is a unique thread in the rich tapestry of human experience.

Embracing sexual diversity isn't merely about tolerance; it's about genuine acceptance and celebration of the full spectrum of human sexuality. It's about creating spaces where individuals feel safe to express their authentic selves without fear of judgment or discrimination.

In every corner of our lives—be it our schools, workplaces, communities, or personal relationships—embracing sexual diversity means actively challenging stereotypes, dismantling biases, and advocating for equal rights and opportunities for all. It means amplifying the voices of marginalized communities, uplifting their stories, and centering their experiences in conversations about sexual health and relationships.

By embracing sexual diversity, we foster a culture of inclusivity, compassion, and understanding—a culture where everyone's experiences are acknowledged and honored. It's a culture that celebrates love in all its forms, respects individual autonomy, and values the inherent dignity of every human being.

As we continue on our journey of self-discovery and growth, let us commit ourselves to embracing sexual diversity in all its beauty and complexity. Let us stand as allies and advocates for inclusivity, ensuring that every individual has the opportunity to live authentically and love boldly. Together, we can create a world where diversity is not just accepted but celebrated—a world where everyone can thrive, regardless of who they are or whom they love.

Breaking Boundaries: Challenging Stereotypes in Sexuality and Gender Identity

In our journey of self-discovery and understanding, it's vital to confront the stereotypes and societal norms that have long dictated how we perceive sexuality and gender identity. These entrenched beliefs often limit our understanding, confine our identities, and perpetuate harmful misconceptions.

Challenging stereotypes means daring to question the narrow boxes society assigns to individuals based on their sexual orientation or gender identity. It means recognizing that there is no one-size-fits-all approach to sexuality or gender expression and embracing the diversity of human experience.

By challenging stereotypes, we dismantle harmful myths and misconceptions that marginalize and exclude. We reject the notion that there is a "right" or "wrong" way to be sexual or gendered and instead celebrate the myriad ways in which individuals express themselves and form relationships.

It's essential to recognize that stereotypes not only harm those who are directly impacted but also perpetuate a culture of stigma and discrimination that affects us all. By challenging these stereotypes, we create space for authenticity, self-expression, and acceptance.

As readers, it's incumbent upon us to question the messages we receive from society, media, and culture about sexuality and gender. It means interrogating the assumptions we hold about what is "normal" or "acceptable" and embracing the complexity and diversity of human experience.

Challenging stereotypes is an ongoing journey—one that requires introspection, empathy, and a willingness to learn and grow. But by daring to challenge these ingrained beliefs, we pave the way for a more inclusive, equitable, and compassionate world—one where everyone's identity is celebrated, respected, and embraced.

Empowering Advocacy: Upholding Rights and Dignity for All

As we navigate the complexities of sexuality and gender identity, it's imperative not only to understand but also to actively advocate for the rights and dignity of every individual. In a world where discrimination and prejudice still abound, advocacy serves as a powerful tool for effecting positive change and fostering inclusivity.

Advocating for rights and dignity means standing up against discrimination, marginalization, and injustice wherever they may occur. It means amplifying the voices of marginalized communities, advocating for equitable policies and legislation, and challenging systems of oppression that deny individuals their inherent rights and freedoms.

Empowering readers to advocate for the rights and dignity of all individuals, regardless of sexual orientation or gender identity, is not just a moral imperative—it's a call to action rooted in principles of equality and justice. It's about recognizing that every person deserves to live authentically, free from fear, discrimination, and violence.

As readers, you have the power to effect change in your communities, workplaces, and society at large. Whether it's through grassroots activism, community organizing, or legislative advocacy, your voice matters, and your actions have the potential to shape a more inclusive and equitable future for all.

Advocacy is not always easy, and it may require stepping out of your comfort zone and confronting difficult truths. But by standing in solidarity with marginalized communities and speaking out against injustice, you contribute to the collective effort to build a world where everyone can live with dignity, respect, and equality.

In advocating for the rights and dignity of all individuals, we not only uphold the principles of justice and equality but also affirm the inherent worth and value of every human being. Together, let us commit ourselves to the ongoing work of advocacy, ensuring that the rights and dignity of all individuals are respected, protected, and upheld.

Navigating Peer Pressure: Making Informed Choices for Sexual Health

In the journey of adolescence and beyond, peer pressure can often exert a powerful influence on our decisions regarding sexual health and relationships. Whether it's pressure to conform to societal norms, engage in risky behaviors, or adhere to rigid gender roles, navigating peer pressure requires resilience, self-awareness, and a commitment to making informed choices.

One of the first steps in overcoming peer pressure is recognizing its presence and understanding its impact on our decision-making process. Peer pressure can manifest in subtle ways, such as subtle comments or expectations from friends, or more overt forms, such as direct persuasion or coercion. By acknowledging these influences, we can begin to assert our autonomy and make choices that align with our values and priorities.

Developing strong communication skills is essential for navigating peer pressure effectively. By being assertive and expressing our boundaries clearly and confidently, we can resist external pressures and assert our autonomy in sexual encounters and relationships. Additionally, seeking out supportive friends and allies who respect and support our decisions can provide a valuable source of encouragement and validation.

Making informed decisions about sexual health and relationships also requires access to accurate information and resources. Educating ourselves about contraception, STI prevention, consent, and healthy relationships empowers us to make choices that prioritize our well-being and safety. Additionally, seeking guidance from trusted adults, healthcare providers, or reputable sources can provide valuable support and guidance in navigating complex situations.

Ultimately, overcoming peer pressure is about cultivating self-confidence, resilience, and a strong sense of self-worth. By prioritizing our own values, boundaries, and well-being, we can navigate peer pressure with grace and confidence, making choices that honor our individual needs and desires. In doing so, we empower ourselves to take ownership of our sexual health and relationships, leading to more fulfilling and satisfying experiences in the journey of adolescence and beyond.

Building Healthy Relationships: Nurturing Respectful Connections

In the tapestry of our lives, relationships form the threads that weave together our experiences, emotions, and identities. Whether with romantic partners, friends, or family members, cultivating healthy and respectful connections is essential for our well-being and fulfillment. In this chapter, we delve into the art of building relationships founded on trust, communication, and mutual respect.

At the heart of building healthy relationships lies the foundation of respect. Respecting ourselves and others is the cornerstone of fostering connections that uplift and empower. It means honoring our own boundaries and values while also acknowledging and validating the perspectives and boundaries of those around us.

Effective communication is another key pillar of healthy relationships. Open and honest communication allows us to express our needs, desires, and concerns authentically, fostering understanding and intimacy. By actively listening to others and expressing ourselves clearly and compassionately, we create a space where trust and vulnerability can thrive.

Empathy and compassion are essential qualities for nurturing healthy relationships. Understanding and validating the emotions and experiences of others fosters connection and empathy, deepening our bonds and strengthening our relationships. By extending kindness and support to those we care about, we create a foundation of trust and intimacy that withstands the tests of time.

In navigating the complexities of relationships, it's essential to set boundaries that honor our needs and values. Boundaries create a framework for respectful interaction, ensuring that our relationships are built on mutual consent and understanding. By communicating our boundaries clearly and assertively, we establish a framework for healthy and fulfilling connections.

Ultimately, building healthy relationships requires ongoing effort, communication, and self-reflection. It's about prioritizing respect, empathy, and authenticity in our interactions with others, fostering connections that enrich our lives and bring joy and fulfillment. As we navigate the intricacies of relationships, let us strive to cultivate connections that uplift and empower, creating a world where respect, love, and understanding reign supreme.

Communicating Consent: Honoring Boundaries and Respect

In the realm of sexual interactions, clear and enthusiastic consent is not just a nicety—it's an absolute necessity. Understanding and communicating consent is essential for ensuring that all parties involved feel safe, respected, and empowered in their sexual encounters. In this chapter, we delve into the importance of enthusiastic and ongoing consent, emphasizing its role in fostering healthy and respectful sexual interactions.

Consent is more than just a verbal agreement—it's an ongoing and active process of communication and mutual respect. It means that all parties involved willingly and enthusiastically agree to engage in sexual activities without coercion, pressure, or manipulation. Consent must be freely given, reversible, informed, enthusiastic, and specific, and it can be withdrawn at any time if one party feels uncomfortable or unwilling to continue.

Effective communication is the cornerstone of obtaining and expressing consent in sexual interactions. It's about openly discussing desires, boundaries, and expectations with our partners, creating a space where both parties feel comfortable expressing their needs and desires. By actively listening to our partners, respecting their boundaries, and asking for consent at every step of the way, we cultivate an environment of trust, respect, and mutual understanding.

Enthusiastic consent goes beyond mere compliance—it's about expressing genuine desire and excitement for the sexual encounter. It means actively participating in the experience, expressing enthusiasm, and demonstrating genuine interest and pleasure. Enthusiastic consent ensures that all parties involved are fully engaged and enjoying the experience, creating a sense of intimacy and connection that enhances the overall sexual encounter.

Consent is not just a one-time agreement—it's an ongoing process that requires constant communication and awareness. It's essential to check in with our partners regularly, ensuring that everyone is still comfortable and consenting to the activities taking place. By prioritizing ongoing consent, we create a culture of respect, trust, and empowerment in our sexual interactions, fostering healthier and more fulfilling relationships.

As we navigate the complexities of sexual interactions, let us prioritize clear and enthusiastic consent, honoring our own boundaries and respecting the boundaries of others. By communicating openly, listening actively, and respecting each other's autonomy, we can create a world where consent is not just a concept—it's a fundamental aspect of healthy and respectful sexual relationships.

Coping with Challenges: Navigating the Bumps in the Road

In our journey of sexual exploration and self-discovery, it's inevitable that we encounter challenges and obstacles along the way. From societal stigma and discrimination to mental health struggles, these challenges can sometimes feel overwhelming and daunting. In this chapter, we'll explore some common challenges that teens may face in their sexual journey and discuss strategies for coping and overcoming these obstacles.

One of the most significant challenges that teens may encounter is societal stigma and discrimination surrounding sexuality and gender identity. In many societies, there are still prevailing attitudes of shame, judgment, and intolerance towards individuals who deviate from traditional norms of sexuality and gender. This stigma can manifest in various forms, including bullying, harassment, and exclusion, leading to feelings of isolation and alienation. Coping with stigma requires resilience, self-acceptance, and finding supportive communities where one can feel accepted and understood.

Another challenge that teens may face is navigating mental health issues that impact their sexual well-being. Depression, anxiety, trauma, and other mental health conditions can have a profound impact on one's relationship with their body, sexuality, and sexual experiences. It's essential for teens to prioritize their mental health and seek support from trusted adults, healthcare professionals, and mental health resources. By addressing mental health concerns proactively, teens can improve their overall well-being and enhance their ability to navigate their sexual journey with resilience and self-compassion.

Additionally, teens may encounter challenges related to sexual health and reproductive rights, such as access to comprehensive sex education, contraception, and reproductive healthcare services. Limited access to accurate information and resources can hinder teens' ability to make informed decisions about their sexual health and relationships, putting them at risk for unintended pregnancies, STIs, and other health issues. Advocating for comprehensive sex education, access to contraception, and reproductive rights is crucial for ensuring that teens have the knowledge and resources they need to make empowered choices about their sexual health.

In coping with these challenges, it's essential for teens to cultivate resilience, self-awareness, and a strong support network. By seeking support from trusted friends, family members, and professionals, teens can navigate the bumps in the road with greater confidence and resilience. Additionally, practicing self-care, setting boundaries, and engaging in activities that bring joy and fulfillment can help teens maintain their mental and emotional well-being amidst life's challenges.

As we navigate the ups and downs of our sexual journey, let us remember that challenges are a natural part of growth and self-discovery. By acknowledging our struggles, seeking support when needed, and cultivating resilience, we can overcome obstacles and emerge stronger, wiser, and more empowered on our journey towards sexual health and well-being.

Final Words of Encouragement: You're Not Alone on This Journey

As we come to the end of our journey together, I want to take a moment to offer you some final words of encouragement and support. Navigating your sexual journey as a teen can be both exhilarating and challenging, filled with moments of joy, discovery, and growth, as well as moments of uncertainty, doubt, and confusion. But no matter where you are on this journey, please remember that you're not alone.

You are a unique and valuable individual, deserving of love, respect, and dignity. Your experiences, desires, and feelings are valid and worthy of acknowledgment. As you continue to explore your sexuality and navigate the complexities of relationships, know that there is no one-size-fits-all approach or timeline. Your journey is yours alone, and it's okay to take things at your own pace, to make mistakes, and to learn and grow along the way.

It's essential to surround yourself with people who uplift and support you, who respect your boundaries and honor your autonomy. Seek out friends, family members, and mentors who celebrate your uniqueness and encourage you to embrace your authentic self. And remember, if you ever feel overwhelmed or unsure, there are professionals and resources available to support you, from counselors and healthcare providers to online forums and helplines.

Above all, I want to remind you to be kind to yourself. You are worthy of self-compassion and self-love, regardless of your perceived flaws or shortcomings. Embrace your strengths, celebrate your accomplishments, and forgive yourself for your mistakes. Remember that growth and self-discovery are lifelong processes, and every step you take towards understanding yourself and your desires is a step in the right direction.

As you embark on the next chapter of your journey, I encourage you to approach it with curiosity, courage, and an open heart. Embrace the unknown, celebrate your victories, and learn from your challenges. And know that wherever your path may lead you, you have the strength, resilience, and inner wisdom to navigate it with grace and authenticity.

Thank you for allowing me to be a part of your journey. I believe in you, and I'm rooting for you every step of the way. Remember, you are not alone, and you are capable of creating a life filled with love, joy, and fulfillment. Keep shining bright, and never forget that you are enough, just as you are.

THE END